How to Make Love to a Woman

69 Orgasmic Ways to Have Mind-Blowing Sex

**By Xaviera Hollander
with Katje van Dijk**

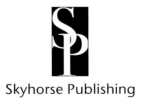

Skyhorse Publishing

Skyhorse Publishing books may be purchased in bulk at special discounts for sales promotion, corporate gifts, fund-raising, or educational purposes. Special editions can also be created to specifications. For details, contact the Special Sales Department, Skyhorse Publishing, 307 West 36th Street, 11th Floor, New York, NY 10018 or info@skyhorsepublishing.com.

Skyhorse® and Skyhorse Publishing® are registered trademarks of Skyhorse Publishing, Inc.®, a Delaware corporation.

Visit our website at www.skyhorsepublishing.com.

10 9 8 7 6 5 4 3 2 1

Library of Congress Cataloging-in-Publication Data is available on file.

ISBN: 978-1-62636-157-7

Printed in China

CONTENTS

Acknowledgments   *iv*

Introduction   *v*

THE BASICS   1

CASANOVA'S DOS & DON'TS   44

POSITIONS & TRICKS   95

GETTING KINKY   146

Epilogue   *201*

ACKNOWLEDGMENTS

My heartfelt thanks and gratitude to Katje, as I could never have put this book together without her. She was my muse, my inspiration, and my organizer. Best of all, we had much fun putting this together. Thank you, Katje, for your hard work, and for lending your sense of humor to the process.

INTRODUCTION

"In my opinion there are really very few frigid women and lots of lousy lovers."
—Xaviera Hollander,
Penthouse Letters, *August 1978*

What I have put together in these pages are the best tips for pleasuring a woman, and in the process, have mind-blowing sex. And if you follow the advice herein, you will have that kind of sex over and over again. I tried hard to avoid doing what others have done—and that is: stating the obvious. You will not find advice in here about how to attract and seduce a mate; you won't hear me telling you to brush your teeth before a kissing session. You should know that already. These sixty-nine tips are devoted to getting you to mind-blowing sex, time and time again. If you want the basics, buy one of those other books. This book is for the man who is serious about getting the most out of his sex life.

I do start by assuming you have a sex partner in your life, because, for most women, the casual dalliance or "one night fling" is not usually where she has had her best sex. It happens, but it is rare. For most women, to get to good sex they have to abandon themselves to the animal act, and getting to that point requires a lot of trust. You can't build the kind of trust you need, generally, in the first date.

Yes, there are couples who report having mind-blowing sex the first time, but I would say that this happened either because they had gotten to know each other very well ahead of time, or because the man had a lot of experience and was very good at reading her, or else they were just both horny as hell and it scratched an itch and seemed mind-blowing, even though it was rather ordinary.

If you want consistently great sex, you must please your partner. If you want her purring at your feet and willing to play any game or do anything your vivid imagination comes up with, you have to keep yourself focused on her satisfaction first and foremost. Great lovers know that. Great sex is unforgettable sex, and great lovers are known for making an unforgettable memory, a memory that remains with her for years or decades to come. That's what you want, and that's what this book will coach you to do.

THE BASICS

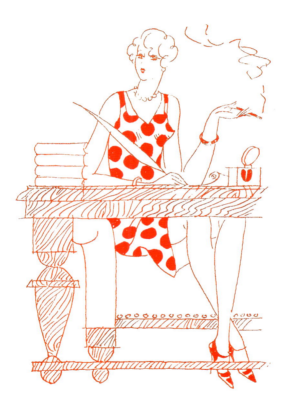

1

UNDERSTAND THE HOLY TRILOGY OF THE CLITORII

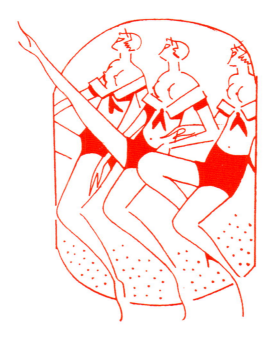

For more than thirty years, I have been advising men that when it comes to women, more than 90% of sex is between the ears. Recently, I had an opportunity to interview a modern day "dating and mating anthropologist" Robert Sherwood. He lamented that the problem with men is that they don't look past the one clit—they don't see that women have three clits. Mr. Sherwood expounded on his theory of the Trinity of the Clitorii. "All three are erogenous zones," he said. "And they are all intricately connected. If you feed only one of the three, or even two of the three, she will starve. You must tend to all of her clits, as if they are one." I was delighted with his metaphor because it put an exclamation point on my theory—you can't just tease the body, you have to tease her mind and heart as well.

Women have much more complex needs than men and a man needs to understand that complexity to be a great lover. You can take all the sex tips in the world, but unless you can read her needs properly, and unless you can apply the actions to her moods properly, you are going to miss the mark and mind-blowing sex will elude you. One woman wants it hard and rough and another wants it soft and cuddly. The same woman will want both at different times. She may need to be taken one night and another time she wants a very easy friend to cuddle with. You have to learn all you can learn about her and then apply it to cradling her heart clit and tickling her brain clit. And, of course, if you don't feed her vivid imagination and need for fantasy, she will likely find someone who can.

Generally, men are much more simple beings. As a group, you have your complexities and issues, but when it comes to matters of the heart, the simpler the better for most men. Here's your tip: Dump that mode of thinking and learn to be more complex yourself. **Learn to present both the good boyfriend and the bad.** "Women are seeking the perfect combination of gentleman and arse," said Mr. Sherwood, and he's right. Get in touch with the warrior and the wimp in you. Seek out the good guy and bad guy in you. And learn how to present each at just the right moments.

> *"Sex is one of the nine reasons for incarnation. The other eight are unimportant."*
> —George Burns

To get her heart clit stimulated, you just have to be a decent person. Have high integrity. Do what you say you are going to do. Say what you mean. Make her feel safe. A woman's heart craves safety.

To stimulate her brain clit, abandon the good boy and bring out the bad boy. Women are genetically programmed to seek out the alpha male (the bad boy) and he is the one who stands out from the pack. It's the same reason why a beautiful woman can have four men fawning all over her and the one she is rubber-necking is the one who just insulted her as he passed by. Well, sort of insulted her. What he was really doing was tickling her brain clit when he leaned down close and said, "You'd be mighty pretty if you didn't wear so much make-up." He made himself stand out from the pack, he stimulated her brain clit by challenging her, and he did it discreetly, privately, which was another signal—this one to her heart clit, a signal that said "this man would be safe to engage with." That's why I said it is complicated. The heart wants safety—the brain wants thrill.

To be a great lover, to provide mind-blowing sex time and time again, you must first understand and come to grips with the Holy Trinity of the Clitorii. You must understand the varying needs of the various clits. You must learn to engage the brain clit, soothe the heart clit, and if you do that, the body clit will follow you in any flavor of sex, any game, any position, any time, any place, and anywhere.

2

GET HER TALKING AND SHARING

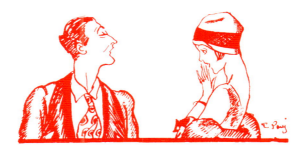

Once I was interviewed on a TV show with Tom Snyder, who asked me what I liked to do best with a new lover. I replied, "It's a four-letter word that ends in 'K,' and it means 'intercourse,' and I like to do it all night and a lot of the rest of the time." Tom said "Oh, I've got my hand ready on the bleeper button," grinning at me. "It's the big one, isn't it?" he asked. "It's big with me," I replied. "The word is 'talk.'"

"Women can be ruined by lovers, but mere acts of libertinism are quickly forgotten."
—Madame Saint-Ange, who claimed to have slept with over 12,000 men during twelve years of marriage

"Intercourse" also means "communication," and if she can't talk to you or you can't talk to her, your experiences of mind-blowing sex are going to be quite limited. The better you communicate verbally with your lover, the better the sex is going to be. Quality conversation is a huge part of sex and, for most women, the key to stimulating the brain clit. It is also the fastest way for you to learn what you need to learn about her so you can do what you need to do to make it safe for her heart clit. Never forget the heart clit: if you don't make it safe for her, she won't go to the limits for you. Her heart clit must be safe in order for her brain clit to go for the gold.

And if you take care of those dominant clits (the heart and brain), the body clit will absolutely follow.

Getting women to talk is not usually a problem, but most women would rather die than verbalize the secrets of their anatomy and they are much worse about sharing the secrets of the dominant clits. Gentlemen, proceed with caution; go slowly, and expect to have to build some trust first.

> *"Basically, I think I was furious with my mother for not teaching me how to be a woman, for not teaching me how to make peace between the raging hunger in my cunt and the hunger in my head."*
>
> —*Erica Jong,* Fear of Flying

And it's quite fair to use every trick in the book, including asking her if she'll tell you one simple fantasy, and if necessary, asking her while her clit is writhing under the pleasure of your tongue. Make sure she understands that the only reason you want to know is because your number one interest is in pleasing her. Withhold cock from her at an untimely moment and make her promise to tell you one little thing, and assure her that you won't ask again for a month. Tend to her heart clit at the same time. Make her feel safe to tell you anything. That's the only way she'll share her secrets. It is highly worth the trouble. Because once you can talk about your fantasies, once you have a trusted and beloved play partner, the sky is the limit and sexual freedom is at hand.

Be ready, though, to hear things that might shock you. One man from a very white suburb in middle America, bought a couples game from the local bookstore, a game which required that he and his wife make a list of fantasies that each of them always wanted to play out. In between "have you wash my hair" and "have you suck on my toes," she had written "Have you watch me do it with a big, angry black man." Mr. Middle America thought she was kidding.

3

BRING ALL THE CONFIDENCE YOU HAVE, ALL YOU CAN MUSTER

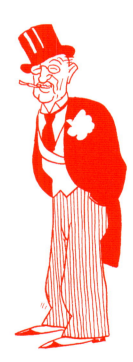

There is probably nothing more unromantic than a bumbler. If you have games you want to play, positions you want to try, places you want to do it, then you must be able to put those into literate sentences. Practice if you have to, but get so that what comes out of your mouth sounds like the most natural and wonderful thing the two of you could do together. If she balks, act like you don't understand. Scratch your head. Say, "Why would you be afraid to do that?" and fall to your knees and say, "Baby, I adore you. . . . I just want to play together."

If you are going to attempt to have mind-blowing sex, you have to have some ideas about how you would achieve that and you have to be able to communicate them, confidently, and with charm. If you can't do the charm thing, then be extra bossy and explain that you can't help yourself, she turns you on so much that you become this whole other animal. Women will cut men a lot of slack for sins made in the name of their beauty.

Even if you are experimenting for the first time, be confident, at least, about how you want to play and what you want to do. Be absolutely OK with who you are—don't apologize for anything about yourself; you have to like yourself if you want someone else to like you, and all men should have figured that out by now.

4

NO COMPLAINTS

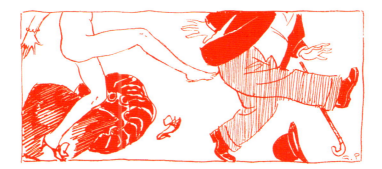

Throughout every interaction leading up to the mind-blowing sex, make sure you do not complain about anything. Complaining is too close to whining and whining is a physical turn off for most healthy and normal women. It is a sad fact that some people seem to find everything in life so unpleasant that they do nothing but grumble. These are the losers of our world. If a person only gets his kicks out of complaining, I say let them—but don't make the mistake of hooking up with one of them. Remember that advice for all your dates. Nothing turns off a person faster than chronic unhappiness and if you can't get through a first date without complaining about someone or something, then you are not likely to have many more.

> *"Having sex is like playing bridge. If you don't have a good partner, you'd better have a good hand."*
>
> *—Woody Allen*

The exception to this, of course, is if your fantasy role-play demands complaints—many of them do. If you are playing the king of the castle and she is playing a low-ly servant girl, then it may very well be a legitimate part of your role to tell her she's moving too slow to quench your thirst, that she should get on her knees to make atonement, and in this particular instance, it's even OK to complain while she's giving you the blow job. Just make sure that when it's over, she has no complaints.

5

NO WORRIES

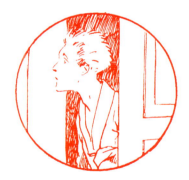

Stop worrying. Worrying has no place in sex—it is an "anti-sex" emotion. When you set out to play, play. Sex is to adults as play is to children and when children engage in a playful activity, they forget everything else and devote themselves to the endeavor. More grown-ups should follow their lead. Lay your worries on the doorstep before laying your partner. Forget the bills, forget the kids, and for goodness' sake, don't go into it worried about your penis size or if you can please your mate.

> *"Man exists in one of two states: getting his dick touched and waiting to get his dick touched."*
> *—Robert Sherwood*

Not that there isn't cause to worry. There is. The male sexual organ is a wayward little prick. A man may find a female irresistibly attractive, but his pecker just hangs its head and ignores her. The next day, however, on a crowded bus or in the middle of a meeting, it suddenly stands to attention for no reason at all, to the enormous embarrassment of the man at the top. This problem is comparatively common in young men and is usually caused by lack of confidence or fear of failure. Unfortunately, it tends to magnify itself because the surest way to stay soft is to worry about not being able to get hard.

The penis is controlled by the brain, and although the programmer of that neurotic computer lives in a bombproof bunker somewhere between the ears, there are ways to reach him. Your dick can usually be coaxed upright by manual manipulation. In the privacy of your room, you can experiment on the kind of caress you like best. I once knew a man who used to smack his cock with the flat of his hand and say, "Take that, you little bastard!" and it would usually spring erect!

6

LEARN TO LOVE YOUR BODY

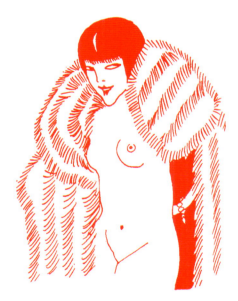

Learn to love your body—or at least learn to pretend! The current environment of "plastic surgery made easy" has people doing all kinds of crazy things to themselves in the hopes of changing their lives radically. By ignoring the fact that one must learn to be comfortable in his own skin, happy with one's own body, many people are missing one of the greatest turn-ons there is in the sexual mating game—and that is confidence. Without it, you are unlikely to experience mind-blowing sex.

> *"There is very little advice in men's magazines, because men think, 'I know what I'm doing. Just show me somebody naked.'"*
>
> *—Jerry Seinfeld*

Sometime in your life, you've seen, I'm sure, the fat, toady, cigar-smoking, roly-poly, bald sixty-ish man walking with a possessive arm around a beautiful young woman (clearly not his daughter), and you probably assume it's a money thing. You could very well be wrong. Women can't resist confidence and a man who feels attractive, whether he is or isn't, emits a powerful karmic aphrodisiac that surrounds him. Men feel the same way about women, becoming hopelessly attracted to someone very average or even ugly, but convinced she is beautiful because she acts like she is. Take a lesson from this.

7

LEARN TO READ HER

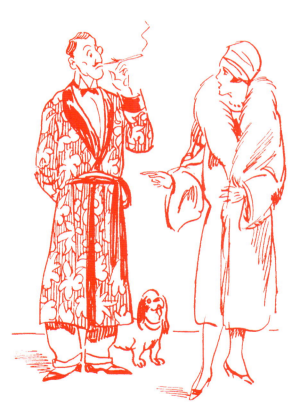

Here's a quote from the *Kama Sutra* that tells you "why" you need to be able to read her:

> "Men who are well acquainted with the art of love are well aware how often one woman differs from another in her sighs and sounds during the time of congress. Some women like to be talked to in the most loving way, others in the most lustful way, and others in the most abusive way, and so on. Some women enjoy themselves with closed eyes in silence, others make a great noise over it, and some almost faint away. The great art is to ascertain what gives them the greatest pleasure, and what specialities they like best."

More simply put, "You must learn to read her, because every woman is different." Every woman's wants and needs are different and you can't be a good lover if you can't give her what she needs, and you can't give her what she needs if you can't read her signals. The signals are always there; few men are good at reading them.

Thirty years ago, two scientists confirmed Darwin's evolutionary theory of emotions that declares that facial expressions are identical all over the globe—that there is no culture where the people express happiness by frowning or sadness by smiling. So there are no tricks here. You just have to be paying attention.

Certainly you've encountered a film where you get a bird's eye view of a woman being mauled by a man she doesn't want to make love to, or a close-up of a woman allowing her husband to make love to her, but she clearly just wants to get it over with. The men in those roles, if you noticed, were not looking at their partners' faces. If they had, they would have known, and they would have stopped.

Good lovers pay close attention to the face and to every reaction a woman's body has to every touch and every word and adjusts his game, if he has to, on his mission to please.

8

STAY FOCUSED

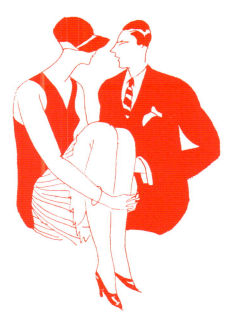

Speaking of keeping your eye on her face, be sure to lock eyes now and again. Don't be afraid to hold her gaze. This "creeps out" some young women—the shy, the inexperienced—but it is also required for many more women. With this latter group, if you can't or won't look her straight in the eyes, you can probably forget about mind-blowing sex. Being able to hold her gaze, to look into the depths of her eyes and see her soul and, all the while, share yours can be a powerfully erotic experience. Don't be afraid to linger there.

> *"The intention is not to leave the body, but to drop into the body more deeply and completely."*
> *—Barbara Carrellas, Urban Tantra*

Eye-gazing is one way to stay focused, to stay in tune with what she is experiencing. Her breathing, what her body is doing (i.e., is she flinching, or pushing into you for more?), her heartbeat, the sounds she is making—this is all information you must contantly be aware of.

9

LEARN TO PLAY

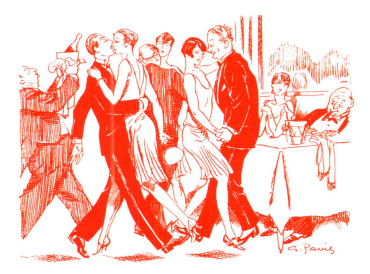

Learn how to play, an absolute requirement for great sex. An ex-boyfriend of mine once told me a story about how he had seduced an actress, who at fifty-something years of age, was still outstandingly beautiful and had a perfect figure. They sat on the couch in her living-room in the presence of her twenty-five year-old daughter, whose boyfriend was also visiting, and pretended that they were a young Victorian couple who were going to elope.

They acted the scene perfectly right up to the final curtain, when they exited and the actress led the way into her bedroom. At that point, the daughter shouted out, "Hey, Mom! Do you want a feather duster to brush the cobwebs off of it?" The point is not the sassy daughter with the delightful sense of humor, but I just couldn't tell half a story. The point is that this man knew how to seduce a woman.

Great lovers are not afraid to look foolish. I think every female falls in love with Kevin Kline in *Sophie's Choice* when he arranges for a picnic where the threesome dresses as wealthy, early twentieth century southern plantation owners. But not all women necessarily like to dress up. Your woman might consider it more erotic to find a place to do some mud-wrestling—which brings you back to understanding her and what turns her on. Sometimes play can happen spontaneously, but if you are not a natural, then do some planning. Think about the type of play she would like and you would like and put some thought into coordinating the event and the timing. It's best if you custom tailor the play to the woman. If she finds it hot to be in hot-tubs, perhaps you engineer a surprise for her that involves a hot tub. Perhaps you fill her hot tub with rubber duckies and let her find them on her own. Or, as another example, if she is very straight, but has an active interest in the goth crowd, perhaps you buy her a wig and costume and make her go out to an expensive restaurant with you as if she dresses that way all the time. The more personal the type of play, the more effective. But all the same, I have included a series of popular fantasy role-plays at the end of the book for those of you who need help getting started.

10

MAKE IT SAFE FOR HER TO PLAY (Taking Care of Her Heart Clit)

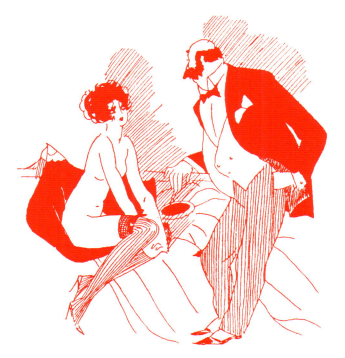

The only way you are going to get most women to abandon themselves to sex, and thereby participate in the "mind-blowing" aspects of it, is to make it safe for her to play. The key to her heart clit is making her comfortable. This is the opposite of how you stimulate the brain clit, but therein you see the complexities of dealing with a woman. You have to learn to make her heart feel safe, so that she will let you tickle her brain clit in unsafe ways. It's required.

I am not going to attempt to explain all the ways to make a woman feel safe, because it would be an impossible task. All women are different; safe to one is scary to another. Some women want to have their hand held every time they go out with their partner, others find this stifling. It's part of your job to get to know her and understand what makes her feel safe.

> *"Emotion is the messenger of love; it is the vehicle that carries every signal from one brimming heart to another. For human beings, feeling deeply is synonymous with being alive."*
> —*Lewis, Amini, Lannon,* A General Theory of Love

Poetry and love letters, flowers and thoughtful gifts, opening doors and steering her gently but firmly with your hand on her elbow or arm around her waist, candlelight and soft music, champagne and a breathtaking view, breaking your stride to help an old woman or a child ... these are the staples of heart clit stimulation. These are the things that make women's hearts smile, but they are not the things that make her wet, not normally. It's the brain clit teasing that makes her wet. But to get there, the heart must be willing and so these time honored traditions remain marks of love and chivalry—easy and not remarkably innovative, and yet consistently effective.

11

WEAR THE RIGHT UNDERWEAR

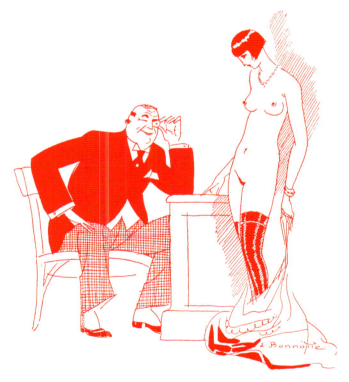

Silky stockings with a seam up the back, high heels, French maid's clothes—these are just some of the clothes that men expect women to wear because it turns them on. And if you heed my advice and you tend to her clits, she will do, say, and wear, anything you want her to do, say, and wear. That's where you want to have repeat sessions, on-demand, of mind-blowing sex. So, find out if she's a boxer girl or a brief girl. If you think these details are unimportant, ask yourself how you feel about making love to a beautiful woman wearing granny panties. Hmm, I thought so. Just find out what her preference is and wear it when you are with her. If the thought of switching from briefs to boxers or boxers to briefs still makes you shake your head, then remember this: I'm not asking you to don four-inch heels.

"I find that slim hipped men tend to wear the briefest of bikini slips, in all different colors. More conservative men prefer to wear white cotton jockey pants. The all-American sporty fellow will like boxer shorts, since they leave a lot of space for his balls to breathe. Of course, the hip young man will wear nothing at all, just so women like me can easily check out his cock and balls."
—Xaviera Hollander, Penthouse Letters, *April 1977*

12

MAKE YOUR SURROUNDINGS EROTIC

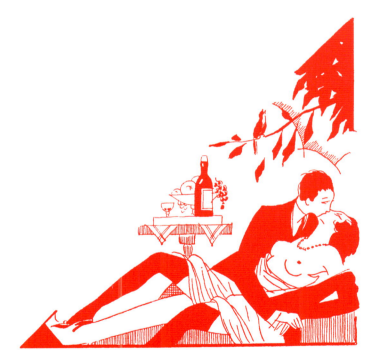

Make your surroundings erotic. If you want to make the statement that you are a sensual being (and who wouldn't want that?) then make sure that where you live has sensual surroundings. Use flowers, candles, soft music, and maybe even erotic art, which today is a field of its own. Feng Shui your way to declaring who you are and what is important to you.

> *"Women need a reason to have sex. Men just need a place."*
>
> *—Billy Crystal*

When you are planning your date, think like a theater producer, like a set designer. Think about what kind of erotic mood you are trying to set and put some energy into adding special touches that will enhance that mood.

> *"Think Like a Set Designer. What is the scene you are trying to create? Is it a Hindu temple? A magic cave? A vampire's lair? Another planet? Be creative! You do not have to go out and have a set built, but keeping an image in mind will make it easier and more fun to choose the elements you'll use to create your space."*
>
> *—Barbara Carrellas,* Urban Tantra

You must know that you have to carefully plan your spontaneity. Only the most practiced and sophisticated seducers can get away without forethought and planning. Scratch that. This group of men has done it so many times that it is habit—which means they are giving it forethought, as well, but without the energy it might take Mr. Average Joe. Women love spontaneity and they don't even mind if it is a bit contrived—in this case, it is truly the thought that counts. Women love it when a man tries to be romantic and tries to be creative. It doesn't happen much, so when a woman stumbles across a man who puts real effort into creating the scene, reading her, and making it right, it is likely she will end up adoring him.

13

TRAIN YOUR BODY

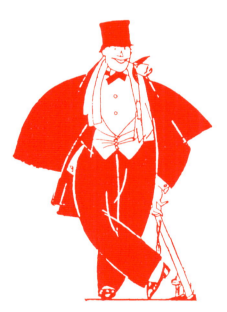

You will never be a great lover without stamina. Men who exercise have more staying power, just like women who exercise have an easier time reaching climax. Maybe it is the act of respecting our bodies, maybe it is the confidence that comes naturally from being fit, or maybe it is purely stamina, but the benefits to your sex life for being in good shape are numerous. Don't try to take short-cuts. Even if Viagra makes your penis stay hard for a long time, if you want to be a great lover, you need to be in shape.

Aside from the physical efforts to get your body to its prime, look also at supplements and foods that might lend a helping hand. There are a number of plants and vitamins, for example, that reportedly help boost sexual stamina. From Linda Sussman's book *Complete Satisfaction*, we get this list of vitamins that contribute to healthy sex: Gingko biloba is known to improve blood flow through the body, promoting potency in men and orgasmic release in women. Ginseng encourages the body to make more testosterone. St. John's wort is a natural antidepressant and a natural libido lifter (it is also known to decrease effectiveness of the birth control pill, so beware on this one). Avena sativa, a green oat straw, is known to alleviate problems of low libido, again, by raising testosterone levels. And finally, there is damiana, which is a sexual stimulant that increases circulation to the genitals.

Sexy fruits and spices known for their aphrodisiac-like affects include oranges, which boost the flow of blood to the penis, and strawberries, which are known for their contribution to sexual satisfaction, Pumpkin pie is said to make both sexes horny (actually, it's the nutmeg and cinnamon, not the pie, but the pie generally comes with whipped cream, and that has possibilities all on its own).

> *"See, the problem is that God gives men a brain and a penis, and only enough blood to run one at a time."*
>
> —*Robin Williams*

Sweat is actually a powerful aphrodisiac. Don't think you must shower after working out and before engaging in sexual activity. Although some clean-freaks will insist, they don't know that sweat is filled with "come fuck me" pheromones. I have read that in Europe during the fifteenth and sixteenth centuries, a courting woman would stick a slice of apple under her armpit and wear it there; when she met a suitable suitor, she would offer him her "love fruit."

14

TRAIN YOUR PENIS

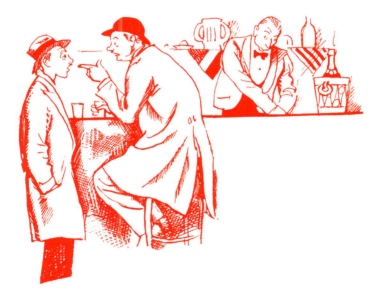

All the truly great lovers I know and have known, were serious jerk-off artists all their lives and they not only regard masturbation as a necessary workout, but use their solitary exercise sessions to practice gaining and losing erections, delaying orgasm, and perfecting new or unusual sexual techniques. In the end, their ladies win from those efforts.

Most men masturbate. Were it not for the fact that there are a few guys around who are genuinely impotent, I would say that all men masturbate. And most men have a complicated two-way relationship between their ego and their penis, i.e., almost all men hate to be caught masturbating. Most of you began masturbating under furtive circumstances, and perhaps, part of the thrill is in the secrecy of it.

> *"The secret masturbator is an addict to his/her solitary sessions and regards them as being on par with religious meditation, a search for nirvana."*
>
> —*Xaviera Hollander,* Penthouse Magazine, July 2001

I once received a letter from a young man that contained a little quiz. It read as follows: Which part of the human anatomy does a man use most when he masturbates? Answer: His ears, as he is constantly listening to see if someone is coming to catch him in the act.

The very horny, and the more intelligent of the male species, masturbate before a first date—to get that tension out of the way, so that he can act normal until the designated hour when acting normal is no longer what the date requires. A normal, healthy young man should, from the age of puberty, have a powerful sex drive—recent studies show that it is normal for them to think about sex every 20 to 30 seconds (the high end) down to a mere few hundred times a day (those with a lower libido). Levels of horniness also fluctuate seasonally, climatically, and according to external stimuli like witnessing the phases of the moon or getting a glimpse of a pair of ladies' underwear hanging in the bathroom.

"People who are scared of sensuality usually end up as campaigners against all forms of eroticism, so if you like sex, and you are in a relationship with one of those, two words for you: get out."
—Xaviera Hollander, Penthouse Letters,
January 1988

Masturbation is simply nature's way of relieving tension; it's also a healthy exercise and the best way to train your penis. In addition, men last longer the second time around and your more experienced female partners know that. Those ladies expect more than one round, and often a mind-blowing fuck requires more than one round.

But sometimes masturbation isn't OK. For years, sexual publications (including my own) have been saying there is nothing wrong with masturbation. Wrong! A man who sneaks off to the bathroom to masturbate as an alternative to having sex with a beautiful, intelligent, caring woman who is panting to make love to him is either asshole of the month or seriously disturbed. On the other hand, masturbation is a perfect antidote to living with an ice-queen and many marriages are surviving only because of the willingness of the husband to take matters "in hand."

One man I knew, who complained that his wife was no longer interested in sex, told me that he took pictures of her while she was sleeping and then slid off to the bathroom and masturbated to those photos. I thought "How marvelous!" because my experience with men tells me that most want to masturbate to fantasies of variety—not to the woman they have easy access to day in and day out. "How cool for her!" I thought, to have a man who kept her front and center of his fantasies. However, one day she caught him, called him a "pervert," and threw him out. I had to advise him that he was better off.

15

TRAIN YOUR BRAIN

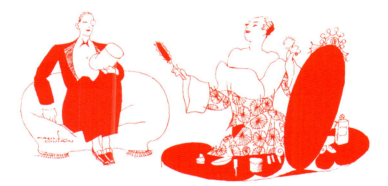

Train your brain through literature and the performing arts. Any man who has not been exposed to these is handicapping himself. Read about love, read the classics—*Romeo and Juliet, Love Story,* or *West Side Story*. Have a decent command of your language. More women are seduced by words than by deeds.

But most importantly, develop your listening skills.

Women are conditioned to believe that men never listen to them. Want to tickle her brain clit? Try listening. And then do that one better. Give her back her own words in a surprising moment. What do most great love scenes have besides sex? Great sex dialogue. And by combining clever dialogue with a bit of surprise (surprise—I was listening!), you have unlocked the key to her brain clit.

Here's an example: In a story she mentions that the waiter accidentally brought her crayfish and she hates crayfish and her story rattles on. You grab at that clue (women drop clues all the time as a result of their chatty nature, you just have to know what to pick up and how to apply it). Hours or days later, you are at a restaurant with her and she goes to the bathroom and when she comes back, you say, "I ordered for you." And she says, happily (she is happy because men don't usually have the nerve to do this, so you've again surprised her), "What did you order me?" And you say (naturally), "Crayfish." And watch her face fall and the smile appear as she gets that you are just messing with her. Humor. Intelligence. You were LISTENING! A triple hitter in the clit department.

43

CASANOVA'S DOS & DON'TS

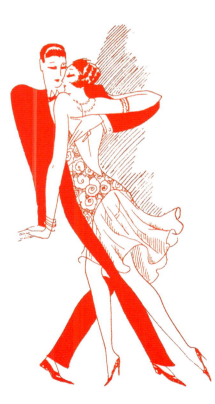

16

DON'T EXPECT HER TO COACH YOU

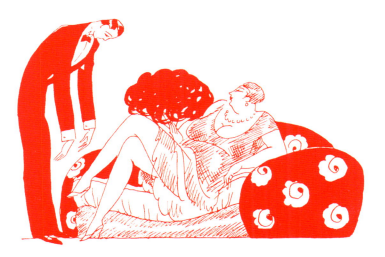

Unless you are a young male hooked up with his Mrs. Robinson, or unless you are on the fringe seeking your dominatrix, you shouldn't be expecting the woman to coach you. One of the reasons women are so reluctant to share their fantasies is because they think you should already know! They don't want to have to explain; they want you to take the clues and signals that she is giving, and work with them. Turn her desires over and over in your mind and come up with something special and suitable to her. That's what she wants. She doesn't want to be orchestrating, managing, or directing. Most women are seeking to be with a man they can trust to do this for them, so, if you want coaching, fess up, tell her you need a Mrs. Robinson, and you might get lucky. You probably won't get "mind-blowing" sex right away—or you might and she won't—but at least you are taking the learning steps.

> *"Many women may want to be dominated but just don't know that they do. Be their teacher, but be absolutely sure that you do your teaching gradually. After all, you don't pick out the handcuffs before you've made the girl."*
> *—Xaviera Hollander, Penthouse Letters,*
> *August 1977*

Confidence is everything in the mating game. Instead of fumbling around and trying to feel the person out, be direct, be clear. And don't be afraid to take the lead. Most women are fascinated by the caveman and his club, much as we bitch about the caveman mentality. It's because unlike the rest of life, it's simple. "He's big, fighting him would be futile, sex will be good anyway, and how fun to not have to think about anything except my pleasure. But he won't think I'm valued if I go at a crook of his finger, so I'll make him chase me around the field a bit."

Women are contrary creatures, but we all have one thing in common—we like to play coy and hard to get. No woman wants to think of herself as "easy," in any sense of the word. If it turns out she wants to take the lead, then I'd say you are a lucky boy and let her, but my experience tells me that it is far more likely that she is watching you, to see what kind of a leader you can be in the game of sex-play—and the game of life.

17

DO USE IMAGINATION, ANTICIPATION, AND SURPRISE

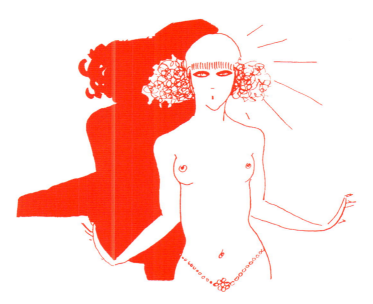

Out in the wide world of working folk, men tend to be more creative than women. But somehow, that creativity dies in the bedroom. A woman, on the other hand, becomes more creative as she ages, as she passes through menopause. If you don't have an imagination, get one. If you have one you are not using, start exercising that along with your body and your penis.

Use your imagination to establish the place, the time, and the theme. Do pick a theme, and you should both dress for the occasion. Even if you dress fabulously every day of the week, there still should be something special about how you are each prepared for a date.

> *"Good sex between good partners always involves some mystery."*
> *—Xaviera Hollander,* Penthouse Letters, *July 1978*

Next, build anticipation for sex by teasing your lover during the day with phone calls, e-mails, or text messages. Make them brief, but to the point—"couldn't wait, had 2 mstrbate 2 thoughts of U," "don't wear underwear 2nite," or, simply, "I can't wait 2 C U."

Studies have shown that women who do mental rehearsals of the pending sex, especially if those women have trouble with orgasms, warm up much quicker than without the preparatory pre-thinking. One study found that the same women who normally required significant physical foreplay to get warmed up, required only thirty seconds if they devoted time to the pre-sex thinking. Part of the return on requiring a dress theme is that it puts her thoughts to sex with you during the hours leading up to the actual rendezvous.

18

DO STUDY SEX TOGETHER

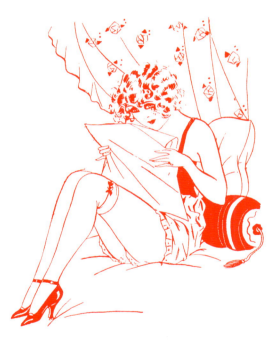

In the process of trying to find out what kind of sex-play would most get her going, engage her in the act of studying sex together. This has the huge upside of providing good sex along the way. You might even tumble upon mind-blowing sex in the process.

Study together. Read the Kama Sutra together. Read erotica to one another; watch erotic films together. A woman who is reluctant to discuss her own preferences will be happy to talk about a movie, and if you are listening, you will hear those preferences in how she reacts to the film.

> *"My general rule of thumb is, if she dresses like a lady, treat her like a slut and if she dresses like a slut, treat her like a lady."*
> *—Damien von Dahlen, advice on how to pick up women*

Be careful in jumping to conclusions though. A friend of mine once told her boyfriend that she thought one of the hottest films out in many years was a film called *The Cook, the Thief, His Wife, and Her Lover*. They watched it together and because there is a serious dose of humiliation dished out to the lead female in the film, her boyfriend—without discussion—concluded that she wanted that and proceeded to humiliate her verbally, in a miserably failed attempt to stimulate her brain clit. She started to cry, then got her car keys and left.

When he caught up with her later, he spent a long time convincing her that he didn't mean any of it and that he was just emulating the husband from the film. As I said, a miserable attempt at stimulating the brain clit.

Here's a useful tip in regard to determining how submissive or how dominant a woman wants to be in the bedroom—and this is just a generalization, but I think it will ring true to your ears as well. I believe that the more subservient the public life, the more she will likely be dominant in her fantasies. Conversely, the more dominant she is in her public life, the more likely she is to play submissive in her fantasies. (This is just a rough guide, boys. You need much more information to know for sure.)

19

DO BRING OUT THE GIRL IN HER

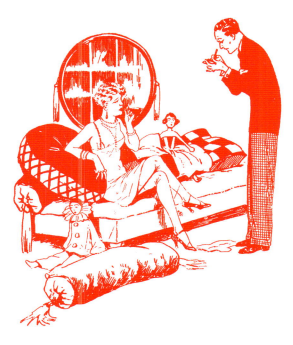

Most educated women today recognize the importance of keeping in touch with their "inner girl," no matter if that woman is 20, 50, or 90. This is important to women, because being in touch with their inner girl keeps them open minded about new experiences, it gives them back a sense that anything is possible, even if everything isn't possible any more. If you want mind-blowing sex, you have to be introduced to her inner girl and she's not going to just offer that up to you—you'll have to search for her.

> *"I would like to have a child. A very wise and witty little girl who'd grow up to be the woman I could never be. A very independent little girl with no scars on the brain or the psyche.... A little girl who said what she meant and meant what she said. A little girl who was neither bitchy nor mealy-mouthed.... What I really wanted was to give birth to myself—the little girl I might have been in a different family, a different world."*
> —Erica Jong, Fear of Flying

So what do little girls like? It's not as hard to figure out as you think. Little girls like laughter and lightness. They like to throw themselves into the act of primping, a form of body worship that begins at a young age. That's a very good starting point for men. Bathe her, wash her hair, paint her toenails, put her make-up on her. Shave her. These are all very intimate acts that tend to revive the girl in the woman.

If your partner is experimental and lets you have a say in her body hair, and if you can't decide whether you want her armpits shaven or not, be bold. Have her shave one and grow the other of her charm pits. A woman would object, but the girl in her would smile gratefully at the idea.

> *"If you men are seeking complete hairlessness, then there is a product designed specially for men, called Golden Balls, available in gay shops in England.... But even if you star in a world-class porn movie, it is still considered perfectly acceptable to have a hairy scrotum."*
> —*Xaviera Hollander*, Penthouse Letters,
> *September 1998*

I have shaved my pussy on many occasions and found that it made me feel like a very horny virgin. And though I have never met a man who didn't adore it, women often object on the very valid grounds that it is a bitch to maintain. In the last decade, however, the pharmacies have started stocking a wide array of shaving tools for men and women, for tender areas and for not so tender areas. The best for private parts, in my opinion, is Schick's new razor with the soap around it, called "Intuition." It's a wonderful little gadget that has the razor built into a square of soap. Years ago I would tell the men, "give her a break, it's not an easy thing to maintain." Now I tell them, if you want her completely bald, then participate in the maintenance, make it fun, and use the right tools.

In fact, you should make a game out of shaving each other. It can be great fun. Even if you are using a razor with the soap around it, don't skip the part about lathering up your partner as a prelude to the actual act. Do it in the bathtub, with you sitting and her standing. Be sure to reach back and get the hair between the front equipment and the ass. Make it more of a game by trying to get rid of all of your own body hair as well, and experiencing complete baldness. A small penis will look much larger with the hair gone and a bald vagina always looks young and innocent. In addition, both partners will experience a totally new feeling of excitement, especially right after being shaved, since the pubic area becomes almost twice as sensitive and even the slightest rubbing of underpants or jeans can arouse you.

20

DO INSIST SHE SLEEPS NAKED

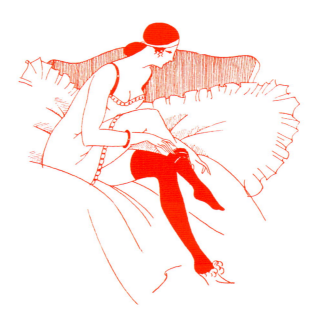

Women aren't the only ones who are bashful about their bodies, but most of the complaining letters I got over the years were from men who wondered why their wives wouldn't sleep naked and actively avoided being seen naked. It's all cultural conditioning and it can be undone over time. Personally, I have no tolerance for digging through night-clothes to get to my lover. I need easy access.

> *"One of the best lovers I ever had was always looking for opportunities to get out of his clothes."*
> *—Xaviera Hollander,* Penthouse Letters,
> *August 2003*

I once had an affair with a Canadian who started off wonderfully naked, but then began wearing a T-shirt to bed. Then one night when winter was setting in, I cuddled up to him to discover he was wearing socks, long johns and a woolly thermal shirt. That was enough for me and I told my lover he could sleep somewhere else because the winters are long, and getting him out of his woodsman gear would be too much effort. But this piece of advice is more about your success than my personal preferences and here's why.

First let me say that if you think that by insisting she sleep naked, you are cheating yourself out of sexy lingerie, you are wrong. Au contraire! The lingerie is necessary and fun, but make sure she understands that when she is under the covers with you, and it is time to sleep, the clothes come off.

You will win on two counts if you insist she sleeps naked next to you and make it a rule from the beginning. Not only will you have easy access to her through the night, but women like the little game of tug-of-war now and again, and the more harmless the game, the more they like it. You are giving her something to wrangle with you about. You are appealing to her brain clit. If she has her nightgown on when she crawls into bed, you say, "What is the matter with you?" and she can then giggle and remove her clothes, or make you remove them yourself. She might tell you it's too cold, clobber you with the pillow and run—in which case, you must chase her! Whatever the result, you are setting yourself up for some steamy sex.

21

DO ENGAGE HER
IN 'DRESS-UP' PLAY

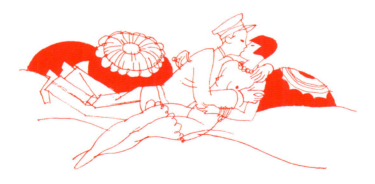

A few years ago, G. Gordon Liddy was interviewed by an Atlanta radio station and when asked the secret to his successful marriage of over thirty years, he answered, "an active fantasy life." If you want to fire up her imagination, if you want to stimulate her brain clit, get some costumes. Get some wigs if you have to. Be willing to don the wig and hook of a pirate. Be willing to be the chef or the police officer. Play different roles with her. She'll say you are insane but her eyes and her actions will tell you that she adores you and she adores the effort you put into the game.

> *"According to a new survey, women say they feel more comfortable undressing in front of men than they do undressing in front of other women. They say that women are too judgmental, where, of course, men are just grateful."*
>
> *—Robert De Niro*

An ex-lover of mine who was raised by British nannies once convinced me to put on the white apron (and nothing else) and simulate doing dishes so that he could get me from behind. Even though I initially resisted, it did lead to mind-blowing sex.

Having intercourse with a nurse in uniform or a doctor of either sex in a white coat is a very common fantasy and fantasy is a great way to get the two of you to the end goal.

I think that the feminist revolution has made most men (maybe just most American men), afraid to tell their partners that they would love to see them dressed in seamed black stockings and a French maid's uniform, or in all black leather, or whatever it is he wants to see. The feminist revolution made being a sex object a bad thing—across the board. So the general male reluctance to elucidate what qualifies as an interesting sex object is understandable. It is a pity, because both men and women are losing as a result.

My advice is that you buy her the clothes you want to see her in. Or at the very least, go shopping with her. And make sure she knows that you will dress in a manner that pleases her, as well. Be sure you don't go on your buying spree before you understand the woman you are dealing with. After all, you don't want to give her a collar if, in her mind, she is the one who is supposed to be collaring you.

22

DO LEARN TO BE AN ACTOR

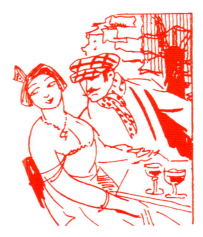

Putting on the costume won't help if you can't let go long enough to put on a little performance. You must get in tune with the actor in you; everyone has one, find yours. She will adore you for it.

One friend of mine had a marvelous lover who could out-act anyone I know. While they were visiting New York City, he told her way in advance that there would be one night that they would separate and meet up in the hotel bar as if strangers. For the days preceding this hook-up, they were forced to avoid the hotel bar because neither wanted it ruined in any way when they finally met as strangers. They didn't want the bartender or anyone in the bar to know they were together.

On the night in question, he approached her at the bar and said, "Susan?" and she shook her head. She was not Susan and did not know this stranger-man. He explained that he had been stood up by his Internet date and that in fact my friend didn't look anything like the woman he was supposed to meet, and struck up a conversation with her and pretended he was a business man with a wife and kids and corn back in Iowa.

When he had her in his room, after they had sex one time and were catching their breath, he admitted to her that he's not married at all, doesn't have a wife or kids or corn, had never been to Iowa, but that he played basketball for some team and had three of his friends in another room waiting to gang bang her. His intent was to scare her. He was trying to present her brain clit with an element of danger. But it backfired because she one-upped him. When he told her sternly of his plans, she giggled and said, "Oh, hon, bring 'em on!"

23

DO GIVE HER THE CHANCE TO "CHEAT"

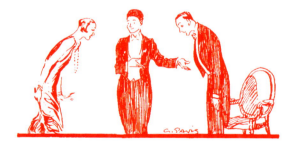

I have heard many stories over the years from people who had discreet affairs and the carry over effect was "mind-blowing sex" with the partner at home. Understand that as women get older, their propensity to cheat increases exponentially. You should be mentally prepared for it.

The current reverence for the MILF* is a case in point. It is so easy today, with the advent of Internet match-making portals, for a suburban mother with three kids and a husband to find "a little discreet sex on the side" (so easy it would amaze you). Young men and middle aged men alike are attracted to the MILF for a variety of reasons.

> " ... the world waited until the end of the nineteenth century A. D. for systematic investigation into feelings and passion."
> —Lewis, Amini, Lannon, A General Theory of Love

Over the years I got many letters from young women starting like this: "Why is he fucking these older women when he could have hot, young me?" When women are young, there is so much urgency to sexual relationships that generally they will engage in sex for fifteen to twenty minutes in silence, except for a few grunts and moans. After orgasm, they bound out of bed and get on with doing something else. That's typical of women in their early twenties.

As women get older and the demands of small children and/or careers lighten up a bit, they begin to understand and appreciate the benefits of spending a whole afternoon in bed with a lover. They begin to relax and open up and by this point in life have gained the confidence to say, "I want to do this or that."

So, the reason why many women, as they get older, as the marriage gets older, cheat is the same reason men do: because they can. And today, thanks to wonderfully robust Internet dating portals, it's not hard for those many under-thirties looking for Mrs. Robinson to find her; nor is it difficult for the married men who might be her age, but are also just looking for some sex on the side.

Women cheat for the same reasons men do, to be reminded of their worth, to show to themselves that they are still desirable to other men. Sometimes women cheat just to experience the newness of a relationship and then they carry that glow home and have mind-blowing sex with their husbands. I know, I get their stories.

For the mature and adventurous couple, you might pre-empt her need to cheat by offering to find and bring a third party home (a man). Another way to provide her with the thrill without actually having to suffer infidelity is to role-play a cheating scene. Have her "act out" to you a confession of cheating and you can make a big scene and perhaps give her the drama she is craving.

*MILF is an Internet dating term used to describe hot women of child-rearing age—"Mothers I'd Like to Fuck."

24

DON'T BE AFRAID TO MAKE "MAKE-BELIEVE" DANGER

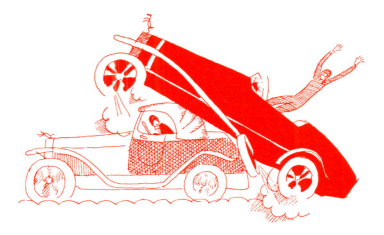

Sex is good, but not worth dying for. I've known people who have sex under very dangerous conditions and, instead, I strongly recommend you simply learn to act at the proper time. Fucking at the wheel is risky, and sucking your girlfriend's nipples whilst peering through the windshield round her female form, however skinny, is definitely dangerous. If that's what tickles her brain clit or yours, then pretend you are driving! Park in a semi-public place and give her a thrill. How hard is that?

> *"Jeeves, the immortal gentleman's gentleman, said, 'I endeavor to give satisfaction.' An admirable quality in a servant, but in a lover one wants more. Passion, pleasure, titillation of all the senses, supreme delight and total fulfillment—these are what making love is all about."*
>
> *—Xaviera Hollander,* Penthouse Letters, *November 1988*

Most women's fantasies involve some danger. The danger makes it exciting. The excitement is what she is seeking. Studies show that the adrenaline rush and endorphins produced from being frightened add to lustiness. Watch a scary movie together, ride a roller coaster together. I have also known couples who have a great time scaring each other with creepy masks, by hiding, by telling frightening stories … and they live lustily ever after, so there must be something to this.

25

DO THINK LIKE A LESBIAN

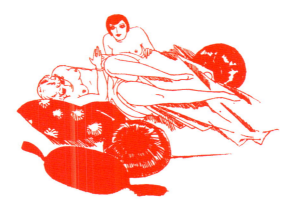

OK, you figured out she likes boxers and you got some and are wearing them. You planned a play-date with a pirate theme and donned the cape and plume. Your dinner was delivered and was in-theme (somehow). The music on the stereo was mellow and, more importantly, to her taste. You are in bed now and it's your turn up to bat with the body clit. Don't dive for it ... yet.

When you get in bed with your woman, try to think like a lesbian. If you've ever watched two women together, they have none of the urgency that usually accompanies male/female sex. They are happy to take a leisurely stroll through the gardens of the flesh and, as a man, you should try to get yourself in that mind set.

You must be willing to do a slow exploration of her body and you will find her erogenous zones. And even if you've been there and done that, do it again! And again, and again.

> *"Women might be able to fake orgasms, but men can fake a whole relationship."*
>
> —*Sharon Stone*

Start your journey by caressing every part of her body and watch her—watch for what she reacts to and what she doesn't. Include massaging the head and scalp as this is excellent pre-foreplay (a relaxant) for many women. Knead, nibble, and squeeze the parts of the arms, the legs, and especially the thighs. Kiss the feet and lick the toes and don't forget to lightly, or not so lightly, spank the ass. Pay attention then, and, when you are through with your journey, you will be filled with wisdom that, applied correctly, will make you a very rich person.

26

DO WAKE HER FOR SEX

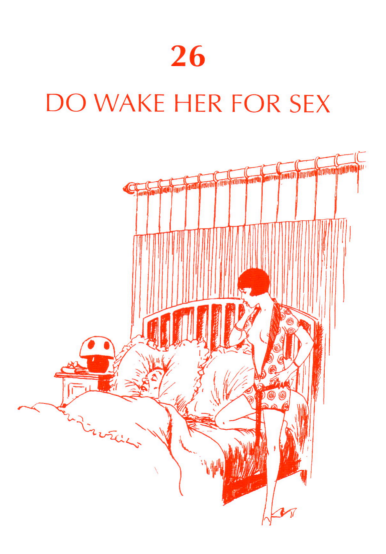

Wake her up for sex. If you haven't woken your lover for sex in the middle of the night, then you are missing something, and so is she. Especially if you went at it earlier, a second round in the middle of the night is very erotic for most women, but choose your timing. She's not going to be so receptive if her alarm clock is set for 6:00 A. M.

> *"Many people who are classified as 'oversexed' are so filled with love for the human race that a beautiful body—and in particular beautiful sexual organs of both sexes—thrill them beyond belief."*
> —*Xaviera Hollander,* Penthouse Letters,
> *August 1998*

27

DON'T LET YOUR PARTNER BE TOO COMFORTABLE

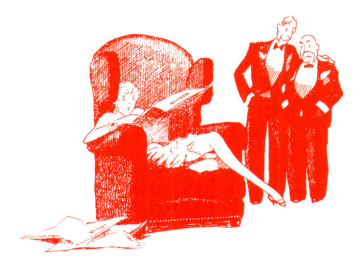

People with a zest for life have zesty sex lives. Boring people generally have boring sex lives. It is sad, but it happens, that we start in a relationship with someone who indeed has a zesty approach to life, but one day wake up and find that he or she has become the latter—the boring person, with a boring sex life, and you find that you have been dragged along to that sad place. If what I said describes you and your partner, you must do something right away! Every day you live with that, you are accepting a second-class life.

A boyfriend of mine had a peach tree which he grew from seed. When the tree was about ten years old, it was beautiful, but had never produced fruit. He consulted his agricultural specialist, an old Spanish farmer, who said, "The tree is too comfortable. Make it feel insecure. Beat it." My boyfriend took a six-foot lead galvanized iron pipe and beat the daylight out of the poor tree. The following season it produced an enormous crop of fruit and has continued for many years. Now, I'm not suggesting that you beat your lover, but there is a lesson here somewhere.

A man never looks so good to his wife as when another woman is noticing him. A woman never works so hard at her relationship (or more specifically, the sexual relationship), as she does when she suspects that her man might be getting bored with her. So, yes, too much comfort and safety can be a bad thing. On the other hand, you don't want to put her on edge unless you are able to do it without threatening her heart clit.

That's not something to be messing with casually. You might take an extra long look at a passing woman, but you better come right around and comfort the heart clit of the one you are with, or the results could be disastrous. The heart clit is the consequential one. The others are much more forgiving.

28

DO STUDY HER BODY

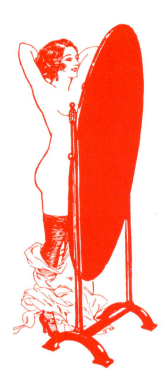

Learn her body as if you intended to sculpt it from memory. Even if some pretend otherwise (or especially if they pretend otherwise), every woman enjoys being with a man who can't get enough of her. Every woman wants to have a lover who is totally into her body. One way of demonstrating how "into" her body you are is by studying it, scrutinizing it—use a flashlight if you think it helps. Make her giggle, make her gasp, and she will protest, but, underneath it all, she will be terribly flattered and likely to reward you in big way.

Try sketching her in the nude. Even if you can't draw well, you can be impressionistic, and flattering.

Use edible body paint for some lighthearted play. Make sure that you are in fact using the edible, washable kind. A woman I knew well was shipped a box of body paints by a friend of hers with a note that said, "Have fun, you two!" and, within a week, my friend arranged a date with her lover for the express purpose of trying out the paints. His daughter was away, her kids were away, and the two of them got naked and got out the paints. Since he is a camera buff, the first thing he wanted to do was to take a picture of her with his name painted across her body. He painted "Humphrey's Property" across her right ass cheek and going down her right leg. He took the photo. They laughed, and he went to get the wash-cloth. Then they learned that it was not washable and the two laughed till they cried over the trick her friend played on them. It took weeks of scrubbing before she got the graffiti off her body. So painting can be fun; just make damned sure it's washable, and, better yet, edible.

29

DO GET HER
TO MASTURBATE FOR YOU

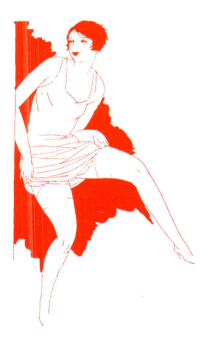

Some men feel very insecure about their masculinity when they see their wife or girlfriend masturbating. This is not the mentality of a great lover, however. The great lovers are thrilled and excited and would pull up a chair and say, "Please, let me watch."

Understand that for the same reasons men like to masturbate secretly, most women don't want to be watched pleasuring themselves. This process, however, can shortcut your learning curve and thus shortcut the time to "mind-blowing" sex.

> *"Saying 'everybody does it' is not the right way to persuade a woman to do anything."*
> — *Xaviera Hollander,* Penthouse Letters, *October 2001*

So insist upon it, whether she likes it or not. Be very patient, tell her how happy it would make you, that you don't like to pressure her, but that you won't give up, and tell her that just the thought of her masturbating turns you on immensely. Negotiate with her, work on her, get her to the point where you have equal rights to her body, and, if you do it in such a way as to make the heart clit safe and the brain clit interested, she will comply.

30

DO FIND HER EROGENOUS ZONES

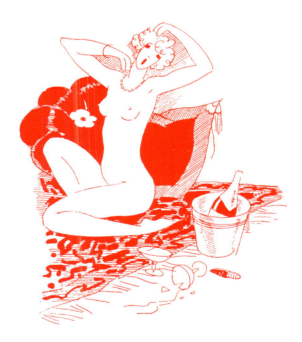

Ears are often an ignored or underutilized erogenous zone. Both the lobe and the area behind the ear are hotwired to the nerves and can be stimulated with a tongue, a light probing finger, or heavy breathing. Some people can orgasm just from ear stimulation, so don't ignore that body part. I sometimes refer to this feeling as an **EARGASM**.

Nibbled with the teeth, titillated with the tongue, the earlobe is a sensitivity center second to none and can be utilized in foreplay with far-reaching results. It is also more readily available in the winter when other, more obvious areas, are concealed beneath layers of thermal clothing.

It's the same with the **neck**. Below the ears, in back where the hairline meets the neck ... these are all erogenous zones. After all, where do you think the term "necking" originated?

Human **hands** have more than 72,000 nerve endings and having someone suck on your fingers as part of the warm-up can be titillating, if part of the exploration process and not a solo act. I once received a letter from a German reader who shared a glove fetish with his fiancée. This couple both wore leather gloves of different types while making love, but they had become so obsessed that they got to the stage of keeping the gloves on most of the time. In their own words, it was like a "superior, second skin."

Unfortunately, the woman had developed a rash as a result, and they asked my advice. Obviously, I told them to leave the gloves off when they were not making love, but I also suggested that they experiment with some "way-out," "kinky" sex, i.e., making love naked. As they were excited by the texture of the leather, I advised them to experiment with oils and creams on their skin (starting off with an ointment to cure the rash). Others wrote me about their "hand fetishes," but I do not classify the human hand as fetish material, simply because the hand is a sexual organ, and as such is used more than all the other sexual organs put together. From the grope on the behind or the grab at the tits, to the delicate caresses, the fingers touching the lips or running through the hair, to the final titillation of nipple or clit, sensation is both given and received through the fingertips.

Hands are sadly neglected as an erotic symbol, particularly in America, where people seem to be more into face-lifts and breast jobs. One can often recognize the true age of a person (male or female) by taking a quick look at their hands, because no matter how well their faces, tits, or peckers have been tightened up, the hand is an area the plastic surgeons have not yet conquered.

The use of nail polish and lipstick go back at least as far as ancient Egypt. Nefertiti appeared to have been a specialist in fondling her lovers' genitals with varnish on her nails, or placing her succulent painted lips around their cocks. The makeup industry isn't making a fortune for nothing out of the sale of perfumes, nail polish, eye makeup, and, last but not least, lipstick. These are the sexual accessories that women smear, spray, or pour over themselves to make them more appealing and attractive to men.

One day, while a group of friends and I were having dinner, we asked one another what appealed to us most about our lovers. One guy said, "I like her dewy bedroom eyes"; someone else was fascinated by his girlfriend's big bottom and matching tits. My own lover told me that what fascinated him about me was my touch, in fact, the way I could excite him almost without touching him. Fortunately, I happen to be blessed with pretty hands—long, slender fingers and tiny wrists, which I suppose I had the good luck to inherit from my mother.

There is nothing unusual in adoring the beauty of a woman's hands, whether she is fondling your cock, loading the dishwasher, or even knitting. Unfortunately, many men do not consider it important to look after their hands. We hear a lot about the delicate, sensitive fingers of a surgeon or a pianist, but never about the square, capable hands of a carpenter or a mechanic. Strangely enough, it is usually men with those competent hands who make the best lovers.

Because of its proximity to the genitals, a woman's **navel** is like a secondary vulva to some men. In the past, women fiercely concealed their navels; now they display them in perfect freedom on beaches and in other public places, in spite of or because of their erotic effect on men.

Stimulating the navel with your tongue, or rubbing body lotion or suntan oil in and around it, can be very sexually arousing to both men and women. Women that have to undergo a heavy stomach operation or receive a cesarean often beg their surgeons to make sure they leave a so-called bikini scar, which is a line that borders on their pubic hair and leaves the rest of their belly untouched and the navel as appealing as ever. Belly dancers often insert a ruby or other precious stone in their navels, and some tribes in India do so as well.

The navel, as well as the crack of the buttocks, is a great turn-on to many men, and, in some instances, an inventive lover has poured drops of champagne in either of these love creases and then devoured the liquid. Tickling a navel with your tongue, slightly scratching around it or teasing it with a feather or a flower or a piece of grass may arouse hidden ardor in your lover.

A little research shows that there is a definite takeit-or-leave-it attitude about this delectable decoration. And when it comes to photo shoots of beautiful women, the navel is rarely featured as a sexual attribute. This is very odd, considering that this beautiful belly embellishment was once so necessary to the erotic paintings of yore.

The incidence of the navel as an erogenous zone seems to vary a great deal, but this also applies to other parts of the body, particularly the male nipple. Very few men are excited by attention to their teats, and, surprisingly, only about fifty percent of women are driven wild by attention to their **breasts**. In my opinion, however, the sensitivity of erogenous zones can be developed through TLC to the extent that one famous lady is reported as saying, "It doesn't matter where you touch me; my whole body is an erogenous zone."

31

DO DISCOVER HER SACRED
PLEASURE PORTAL

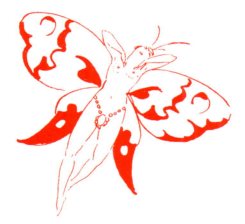

Contrary to popular myth, a woman's clit is not a magic pleasure button. Just as every woman is different, the size and appearance of each woman's clitoris varies. What's more, most of it is inside and not readily visible. It is sensitive and for many women, unless you touch it very gently, touching causes pain; so boys, don't assume that it's a genie's lamp and that, if you rub it hard enough or long enough, you'll get an orgasm. Touching it the right way, for that particular woman, is what is required. I highly recommend that you ask her to let you watch her do it first, especially if you are new to it.

According to the dictionary, the clitoris is "a part of the female genitalia consisting of a small, elongated, highly sensitive erectile organ at the front of the vulva, homologous with the penis." The word actually comes from the Greek word meaning "to close," although another Greek anatomist says it was named for the Greek word for "key" (as in key to pleasure), proving only that, right from the start, we had men classifying something they knew nothing about.

The entrance to a woman's vagina is covered by two pairs of vertical lips, and the inner lips (the labia minora), join at the top in shape of a wigwam, without the sticks. This is the female equivalent of the head of a man's penis and though it is a lot smaller, it has more nerve endings.

In its normal relaxed state, it can be supersensitive, almost painful to the touch, or totally unresponsive. Not only do all women react differently to having their clitoris touched, but the same woman will act differently at different times. Most women require a longer warming up period than men do and in my case, I need kisses and caresses before I'm ready to let a man finger my clit. Sometimes after a period of subtle sucking, my clit cries out for more rigorous attention. Those of you who are new to clit play, proceed with caution and pay attention to your lover's responses. Learn from them.

> *"Although I dislike the predatory aspect of deflowering as many virgins as one can, there's nothing wrong with an older, loving person showing a novice a few tricks regarding getting laid. We tend to teach our young people everything except how to screw."*
> *—Xaviera Hollander,* Penthouse Letters,
> *November 1977*

A good lover will take the time and energy to explore his woman's body and learn all the sensations that rock her boat. Most men will discover her G-spot during the journey. If that's not enough help, however, do this: Wet your fingers with saliva or a water-based lubricant and insert two fingers into the vagina. Touch the posterior wall with your index finger. The sensation of putting pressure on that back wall is often enough to get a woman going. Talk to her while you are doing it and pay attention to her responses. There will be some women who find it uncomfortable (in a bad way) and, if that is the case, move on!

You will know that you are at the G-spot because the skin there feels differently than the rest of the lining of the vaginal walls. The G-spot feels like a small area of wrinkled skin, where the rest of the lining feels taut. Once you've located it, move your fingers around, caressing the spot. Tickle it. Make the "come here" motion with your finger, a sort of scooping motion. You can also use the other hand to stimulate her clit, or use your tongue. Most women really get off on the combination of fellatio and hand-stimulation of the G-spot.

Pleasurable vaginal play depends on moving slowly to generate fairly symmetrical sensations, and remembering that the border between pleasure and pain here is razor thin. A man should get to know the size and shape of his partner's vagina, and remember that it changes shape depending on where she is in her menstrual cycle and how excited she gets.

Be aware that problems for women reaching orgasm can be physical in nature. Beware of hooded clitoris syndrome: A little foreskin over her clit could be preventing her from feeling sensations she would otherwise experience. If this is the problem, the covering can be surgically removed and the problem will no doubt disappear along with the extra skin. If the problem lies elsewhere, it won't be so easily remedied. I hate to suggest that one use alcohol to enjoy sex—drinks just help to deaden certain erotic possibilities—but some women might need a little alcohol just to help over-come inhibitions. Also, you may be placing too much emphasis on her having an orgasm. It isn't everything, despite what a number of sexologists say. Sex can be great without orgasms. Don't get me wrong—I love my orgasms, but it doesn't always have to end with a big bang.

For the more adventurous couple, here's a tip I love from howtohavegoodsex.com, a great source for matters of the female body: Using your index finger and thumb this time, pull together some of the tissue from the vaginal walls and rub it together using the fin-ger and thumb. Start out very carefully and very gently and pay attention to her response. If you are causing irritation or she just doesn't like the feeling, move along. However, many women have been driven up the wall by this, so it's worth a try. Remember, it is better to err on the side of too soft, rather than too hard, as too soft isn't likely to end your play but causing pain will. Al-ways give her two different sensations at the same time and then ask her which she likes better. It is easier for women (or anyone, for that matter) to answer a ques-tion if it is simple: "Do you like this?" … "Uh huh." … "Or this?" … "Uh huh." … "But which?" … "Uh huh." Be ready for that. She just might like it all.

Take care not to lose that bear! The vagina is the center of a woman's physical universe and is both mys-terious and magical. New lives begin there. Men spend the rest of their lives trying to return there. Some men have no limits to the experiments they will perform on their women, and some women have their own fetishes for putting strange things up there. Hospital records will tell you that emergency rooms have extracted some pretty bizarre things from the wombs of visitors. The most astonishing I've ever heard of was a woman in New York from whom they removed a stuffed Paddington Bear, complete with Wellingtons, rain hat, and mack, leading one to gasp and left unable to decide if the gasp is in horror or admiration!

POSITIONS &
TRICKS

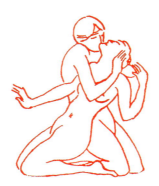

32

ON TOUCHING—FIND HER RESILIENT EDGE OF RESISTANCE

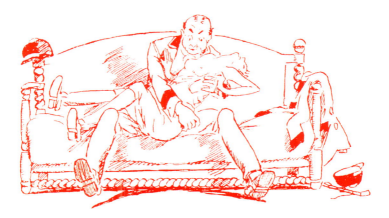

I highly recommend the reading of *Urban Tantra: Sacred Sex for the Twenty-First Century*, by Barbara Carrellas, as it is rich with information on all aspects of sexuality, from defining the relationship between your chakras and your sex drive, to providing sexual rituals and breathing techniques, to dispelling the most common myths of BDSM, to showing you how to make sexual magic! Her book makes most discussions of sexuality look positively one-dimensional.

I often wondered how I could describe in words, to my readers, how to touch one another, especially the first time around, when reading her face is all you can do because the opportunities for discussion are yet to come. I've had novices ask me, but putting in words the lessons surrounding the sense of touch is not an easy task. If you are lying in bed next to your partner, she can take your hand, put it where it feels good to her and even control the fingers, emulating what she would do to yourself. "Showing" I can do and have done and will continue to do, but "telling" is a bit tougher. So when I read what Barbara had to say about the "Resilient Edge of Resistance," I thought, "Bravo—she nailed it!"

From *Urban Tantra*: "When you touch the body, you want to touch deeply enough that the body pushes back just a little. If a muscle becomes rigid under your touch, you've gone too far. If the muscle feels flaccid, you haven't gone far enough. **Sex that is too soft is vapid; sex that is too hard is assault**. We want to learn

97

to dance on the Resilient Edge of Resistance because that's where the real pleasure is. When we reach that level of pleasure, gateways open to even more profound discoveries and connections."

Touching is a matter of feedback—touch first, read her reaction, adjust, touch, read her reaction, adjust—don't forget tip #7 for your "reaction input," and do it frequently. Ask yourself if you are someone who is capable of dancing with a woman at her Resilient Edge of Resistance or do you just kind of plow through the act of sex without incorporating the feedback signals she is giving you? For great lovers, touching is a feedback circle. Touch, measure the satisfaction she is getting—if none, try another way, if some, try a little more ... great lovers never stop measuring their own success in bed—and they measure it by their partners' reactions.

33

VARIETY IS AN ESSENTIAL INGREDIENT

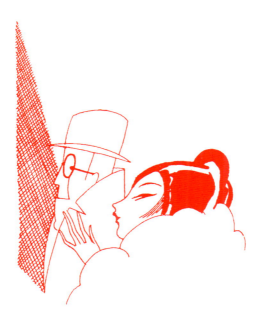

To tickle her brain clit, the essential ingredient is variety. Making one small change in how you make love or seduce will have a thrilling effect. If you do one thing differently than you normally do, your partner will generally find it erotic.

What follows is a series of my most recommended positions and tricks. But remember that most women are easily stimulated by variety. Remember also what you learned about touch and dancing at her Resilient Edge of Resistance. Think about these things when you read the positions and tricks that follow. Some women will love them and some women will hate them and the same woman might like a particular position or action one day and abhor it another, so don't try these until and unless you have mastered the whole business of reading her.

34

UNDER THE WATER

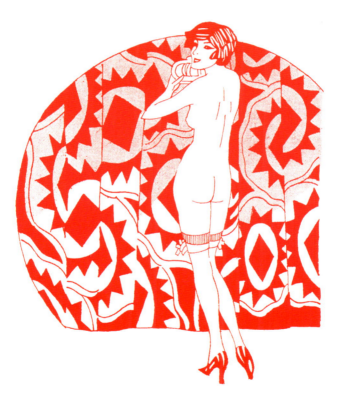

Some places that seem like they might be erotic aren't. Water does have a tendency to shrivel up the penis. Also, even if you manage to maintain a hard-on, the water will make it twice as difficult to enter the vagina. Water tends to tighten up the vagina and makes the entrance rather dry.

I once attended a nudist camp where the men would joke, "Oh look, the water is that cold," and with their fingers they would measure from an average six inches to a tiny two or three. Of course, they were indicating how their cocks reacted to the cold water (shrinkage).

The next time you want to make it in the water, forget about the lake or sea. Instead try screwing her in the bathtub. With the aid of the warm water, some bath oil, and a good bar of soap, you shouldn't have much trouble. You just have to be a bit of an acrobat to find the right position. She can always place herself on top of your penis while you lay back like a pasha.

Also try pleasuring her with a faucet and running water. There are many ways to masturbate using household items, and I've found that each different item produces a different type of orgasm, from the most intense to the most relaxing. My parents used to have an old washing machine that jumped around when it hit the spin-dry cycle. While I was still living at home, I used to turn it on when everyone was out of the house, and, if I leaned on it in just the right position, I could have a fantastic orgasm. I have also enjoyed many relaxing orgasms under the faucet, but for this I find it easiest to lie down in the bathtub while the shower is on. The position is more comfortable and the flow of water is lighter.

If you find the bathtub too difficult to negotiate for both of you, then get the shower going, or run some bath water, get out some toys, position her either on all fours or on her back, and tease her while she is in the tub and you are not. Use the scene as a starting point and you can make your way back to bed for the grand finale.

35

YOU "KNEAD" THAT VULVA

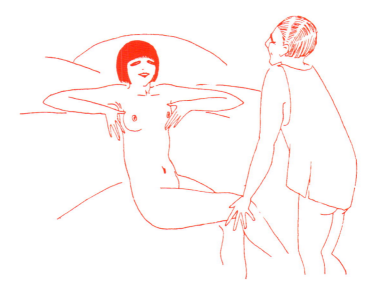

You might begin by massaging her thighs and nibbling gently on her nipples (actually, gently or not so gently, depending on where her edge of resistance lies), but none the less, don't just dive for the clit. Don't skip the preliminaries. Use words too ... you might whisper in her ear that you want her to lie very still because you are about to explore her for real. You might position yourself sitting Indian style between her legs so you can use your hands, see her sacred portal, and see her face at the same time.

> "The certain signs of a genuine female orgasm are twitching of the inside thigh muscles, flowing vaginal juices, and her nipples should be erect at the moment of orgasm."
>
> —*Xaviera Hollander,* Penthouse Letters, *December 1987*

Put the sides of your palms up against the sides of her two labia and smoosh them together gently, and then harder, finding her edge of resistance and responding to it as you must. Then release and repeat—if she responds favorably. Release and move on if she doesn't. Taking your thumb and forefinger from each hand, spread open her lips, sliding your fingers in the groove between her clit and her vaginal lips. Whisper to her that she has a beautiful cunt and ask her again to lie still.

Don't be afraid to massage the area, as the muscles are rather hardy. Remember that the clit is extremely sensitive and so licking and playing with the area around it is often enough a bit painful ... many women will snap their legs together if you do a frontal assault on the clit before it is ready to be touched. And many women will orgasm without ever having their clit directly touched.

It's much more of a turn on to a woman to have a man whispering to her during the act, or giving direction, than to hear grunting and groaning. There is an element of control, I suppose, that a woman is seeking, and though many women want to lose control and grunt and scream, they want a partner who is consistently in control of himself. Excessive moaning or grunting or shouting out "Oh baby, oh baby!" through the whole thing, is not a turn-on for most women.

36

TRY A STOMACH MASSAGE

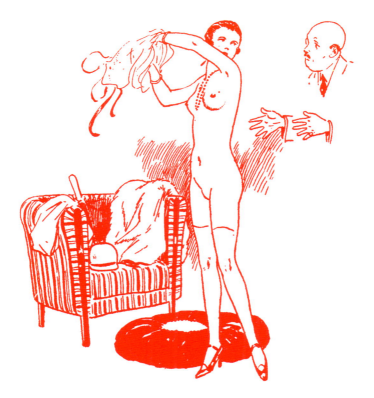

If you have a reluctant sexual partner, try warming her up to a belly orgasm. Either while she is sitting on a chair in front of you and you behind her, or with her on the bed and you kneeling over her, place your hands in a triangle position over her abdomen, and begin to gently massage; again, whisper to her. Ask her to breathe deeply and be still. Continue the massage. A belly massage will titillate the ovaries and stimulate her sexual appetite. Move your hands along, smoothly up her body ... gently squeeze and pinch her nipples, spread her legs and insert a finger to see if she is getting wet ... touch, read, react, and start all over. Soon she will be begging you to let her get up and join you in bed.

37

USE YOUR FINGERS

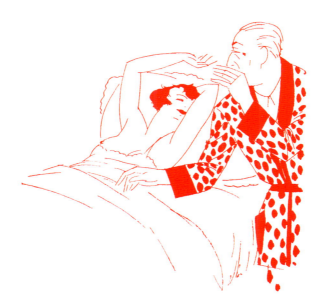

By keeping together the pointer finger, the middle finger, and the ring finger while gently caressing the clit, you will be able to cover a lot of nerve endings at the same time. Linda Sussman calls this "the three finger caress"; I had one lover who could make me come very quickly by employing this technique, but I just called it "that clit teasing thing you do with your fingers."

> *"Don't be annoyed at women for faking orgasm. If for some reason we women fail to have an orgasm at the prescribed moment, it is so much easier to fake one that it is to deal with the series of 'No, I didn't, darling, but it wasn't your fault ...' and all the other ridiculous conversation that will inevitably follow."*
> *—Xaviera Hollander, Penthouse Letters,*
> *April 2001*

Another favorite trick of mine is what Barbara Carrellas calls "The Twist and Shout." Use two fingers and insert them in her vagina tips down and then while you have your hand inside of her, you flip your wrist and hand so the fingertips are facing upward, then repeat twisting right, repeat twisting left.

Most women will enjoy some form of either of these tricks. Remember that whether you are using your fingers or your penis, some women like hard thrusting and some women don't. Most women will happily overlook a size-challenged penis if the man is good with his hands. Hands are important. What you do with them is important. Knowing specific tricks is less important than knowing how to explore, and how to read her so that you can pleasure her in a manner that is desirable for her.

38

HEAD TO TOE AND TOE TO HEAD

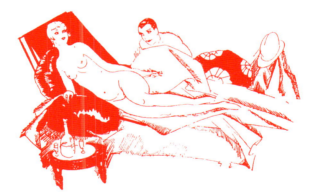

From the website howtohavegoodsex.com, comes this challenging position: instead of assuming the missionary position, where the couple is head-to-head and toe-to-toe, one person should reverse their position, so that the two of you will now be head-to-toe and toe-to-head. Each person has a view of the other person's feet. The angle of entry is not what most couples are accustomed to and it requires the party on the bottom to arch the pelvis and requires the woman to be willing to guide your penis into her vagina. If you can't make it work, don't fret. You will probably get some much needed comic relief as your reward for putting in the effort—for trying something new.

P. S. While each of you is facing each other's clean toes, why not have a nibble? If she doesn't like it then you might want to try an alternate approach: use your hands and massage her feet.

39

ADD VARIETY TO YOUR "QUICKIE"

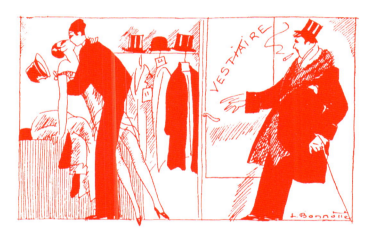

There is a big difference between a "quickie" and a "slam-bam-thank-you-ma'am." The latter is the label women use when a man is a lousy lover and puts no energy into pleasing her. The former, however, is often reported by women as a badge of honor: "I wouldn't have been late if my husband hadn't wanted a quickie before I left." (She sounds like she's complaining, but really she's bragging.) A "quickie" can be a very erotic event, as long as quickies aren't the only thing on the menu.

Quickies occur most frequently in places where there is no access to a bed ... quickies happen in bathrooms, while a crowd is gathered in the living room singing Christmas carols, in the garage, while the kids are playing basketball around the corner, in the office closet at work.

To most men, there is no trick or skill to "getting a quickie." It's as natural as jerking off. It can happen in virtually any place and in any position, but the most common, I suppose, is where the woman bends over the sink, the desk, or the back of a sofa, or uses a chair to anchor herself in some way, and he assaults from behind. (This doesn't mean she gets it "in the behind," although, as I said, "any position," so that happens as well.) Normally, however, it is a vaginal entry with her secured and bent over and him unzipping, inserting, and doing a lot of pounding before the two parties put themselves back together and join the others to face the music, so to speak.

You can add variety to your quickies by taking her face to face, standing up, against a wall (surely you've seen this on TV and yes, you have to have muscles to do this), or by putting her over your lap and bringing her to orgasm with your hands only, paying attention to stimulating both her vaginal and anal entryways.

40

PUT HER ON TOP

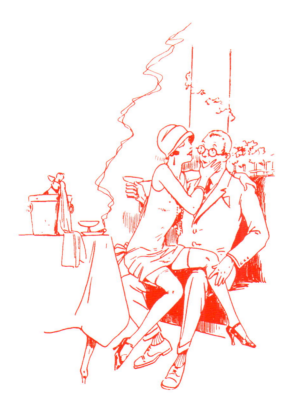

Woman on top is recommended for women who have trouble reaching orgasm or for those who are new to sex, as it puts them in control of the rhythm and depth of penetration. The man can still grab onto her ass or waist and thrust, but she is in a position of control and can find her own way to pleasure. (Warning, although many women like this position, most like it for offering variety, and like anything else, done alone or as a mainstay makes it boring. And this position can discourage brain clit stimulation for those who might not want to be in control.)

Encourage her to tilt her hips back, as this is an angle of maximum pleasure for her. From on top she can also stretch out flat with her legs extended over yours, or she can squeeze her legs together inducing orgasm. She may sit straight up and slide up and down. Many women report that they really like this position because of the added genital stimulation (the vulva rubs up against the man's pelvic bone). In addition, men (again, if they are coordinated) can stimulate their partner's vulva (and/or breasts and/or other body parts) with their hands and women can masturbate themselves easily from this position.

If she is reluctant about getting on top, tell her it's all about watching her and what a turn on that is for you. Actually, this tip works across the board. Positive reinforcement of pleasurable sensations/movements is a good way to encourage your partner to continue doing the things you like her to do.

41

THE DELIGHTS OF DOGGIE STYLE

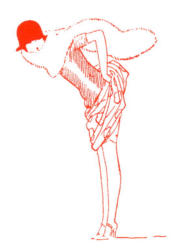

Whenever the man enters the woman from behind he has the unique opportunity to incorporate use of his hand(s) to achieve a multitude of sensations, each intensifying the other. Whether penetrating anus or vagina, having her back against your chest offers you the freedom to explore her other body parts manually. Kneeling down on all fours, or bent over a chair or bed, all variations lend themselves to at the very least toying with her clitoris and surroundings. If both hands are available, the other can be massaging breasts and tweaking nipples. So, guys, if you dislike neglecting those yummy possibilities as much as I do, grab for them!

For variety, ask her to spread her legs very wide—this allows for greater penetration on your part. This will also have the effect of making you feel well-endowed, whether you are or not. If you are indeed a bit large for her and your entry causes pain, then instruct her to clench her legs tightly together as this will have the opposite effect and it will lessen her pain.

Many men like to move from this position to anal entry and that's OK, but don't move from anal to vaginal without stopping to clean up. And don't enter anally without plenty of lubrication. I said I wouldn't state the obvious, and I just did, but on behalf of many bottoms around the world, I feel I must.

42

STIMULATE HER A-ZONE

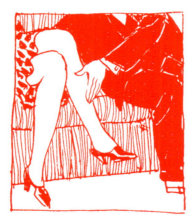

Between the G-spot and the cervix sits the Ahhhhhh Zone (A-Zone) or the anterior fornix zone, as it is scientifically named. It has only been discovered within the past fifteen years by scientists who were investigating solutions for vaginal dryness. Where the G-spot feels spongy to the touch, and the cervix feels like a small round indentation, the skin between the two is taut. When you find it, tickle it. As you are searching for it, be careful how you press against the cervix as pressing too hard can be painful to your partner.

As you are exploring and finding these special places within the sacred portal, be sure to remember that the object is to dance with her at her Resilient Edge of Resistance. Watch her face ... keep your focus ... touch, read, adjust.

43

DON'T BE ANAL ABOUT ANAL SEX

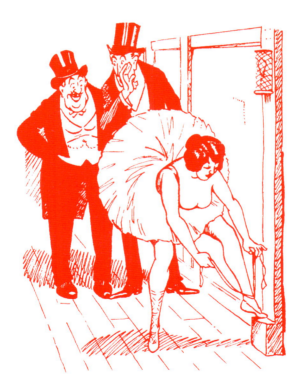

In certain American states, anal sex is still considered a form of perversity and there are laws whereby a married woman can successfully sue her husband for divorce if he buggers her. In this day and age, I find that a bit unbelievable, but it is true! Luckily, more of the states have seen common sense and have revised these antiquated laws in the past quarter century.

Getting it "up the butt" is a supreme act of submission for the buggeree and a supreme act of domination for the bugger.

Anal sex can make even the smallest penis feel huge. And even though there are a lot of people who enjoy taking it that way, there are as many that automatically clench their butt cheeks in fear and disgust at the thought. Fear of the pain, disgust that you even want to put your penis there.

It's probably not so wise to try performing anal sex on a first date, nor is it something you want to wake your wife for in the middle of the night. Better to try some more common kinds of sex-play in those circumstances.

When the time is right, start her off by using your fingers to stroke her ass, kiss her there, perhaps, nibble at the luscious curve of her butt cheeks surrounding the area. Try holding her down with one hand and using your forefinger of the other hand, diddle a while on the outer rim.

If she responds favorably, then try positioning your hard-on against her back hole. If she moans and groans, I'd say you are in luck, but please, please, gentlemen, make sure you are lubricated before you enter. The anus does not have the natural lubricating juices of the vagina. If you're stranded without a drugstore in sight, good old saliva will always work.

"Lubricants (lubes) can be lots of fun, try the flavored brands to enhance oral sex. If you're going to insert something into someone, you should only use a water-based brand. ... Never use oil-based lubes (like Crisco or Vaseline); they weaken latex condoms, dental dams and gloves, making them more likely to break."
—*Xaviera Hollander,* Penthouse Letters, *July 1997*

While you insert your lubricated erection it is best to massage her breasts and clitoris. The excitement will take her mind off any sensation of pain. The best positions for anal sex, from my own experience, are to have the woman lie face down, with a pillow underneath her stomach, or to have the man lie on his back so that the woman can straddle his crotch. The latter position is best at the initial attempts, since the woman controls the rate of insertion. If things get a little rough, she can pull off with ease.

Anal sex may be somewhat painful for the novice female, but then losing your virginity vaginally is also painful. Your more experienced female mates are into reliving the pain of that original experience and so are likely to be more open to it than the novice.

Anal beads aren't for everyone, so remember that when you try them. Also, remember that timing is everything. You don't just shove them up there and yank them out. They are meant to enhance the orgasm, and so the right way to use them is to wait until your partner is almost at orgasm, and then begin to pull them, so that they pop one by one, in a slow rhythmic manner. And if your partner says it hurts (in a non-erotic way), which some people report, then don't use them again. There are plenty of other things to do.

44

THE DOUBLEHEADER

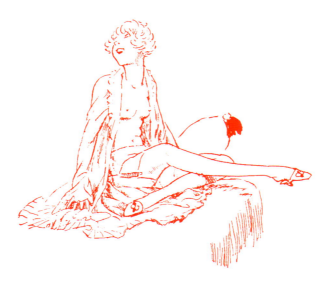

Try the doubleheader; you might like it, too. It started when one of my lovers complained that when I came while we were sixty-nining, I would stop everything and just float away on a wave of pleasure, leaving him hanging on the brink, as it were. Sometimes he would stop what he was doing to yell, "Hey! What about me?" to which I would gasp, "Don't stop, don't stop!" We, or rather he, finally solved that one by stopping, but immediately replacing his tongue with his cock, which he did so rapidly that we hardly missed a beat. This led to what I now call a "doubleheader," a simultaneous double orgasm for me that no one who has not experienced it can possibly imagine: marvelous!

> *"There is a powerful Tantric principle: 'three strokes for thirty.' It is better to make three delicious strokes precisely at the Resilient Edge of Resistance than thirty strokes that are sloppy and unconscious."*
>
> —*Barbara Carrellas*, Urban Tantra

45

VARIATION ON MISSIONARY

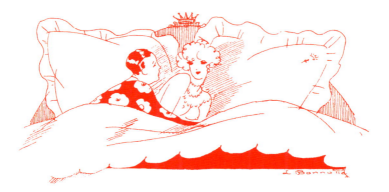

A typical progression of positions during initial love-making between a man and a woman generally goes like this: The man on top, the woman on her back, beneath him—this is the classic and where most people stay during their first round of love-making. There is enough newness, there is the enjoyment of kissing and touching and exploring a new body; it's a time-honored starting point for lovers. This then becomes modified as both partners lie on their sides and continue to make love from a new angle. Then comes doggie style as he takes her from behind, and, finally, a sacred Tantric position, both lovers in a seated position, face to face, he is sitting "Indian style" and she is mounted on top of him with her legs wrapped around your back. These are the four basic lovemaking positions.

In the first position, where the woman is on the bottom and the man on top, if you tell her to pull her legs tight together once she is near orgasm, she may be able to induce the timing of her own orgasm and find a trick she may want to repeat now and again. Doing this will also prove useful (pleasurable) to her if you have a size-challenged penis.

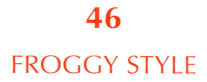

46

FROGGY STYLE

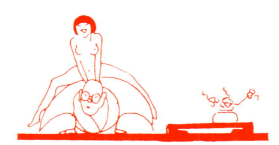

The best position is an extension of the doggie style that I call froggy style, and it is best done on the floor, rather than the bed. The woman bends from the waist and puts her hands on the floor. She bends her knees some, but has her weight on her toes. He is in a similar position, hovering over her. He grabs her cheeks and spreads them and inserts his penis into her vagina, then rocks up and down on his toes causing stimulation to both.

47

POUNDING ON THE SPOT

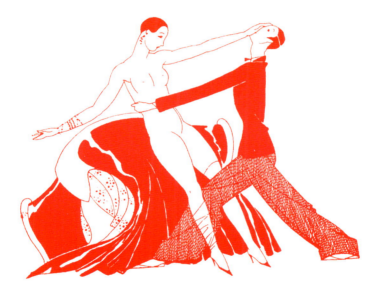

Plain old rapid pounding has been given a bad name by those who do that and only that. The fact is, most women like a good pounding if it's not alone on the menu and if the timing is right (meaning, hot hors d'oeuvres have been served up already). The act of "dok el arz" (Ancient Arabic for "pounding on the spot") done in a particular rhythm is desired by most women and, in fact, for many it is a required course at some point during the lovemaking session.

It isn't necessary to climax at the same time—some people are so intent on ensuring a perfectly timed dual climax (his and hers) that they miss all the fun. As long as both of you are satisfied in the end, that's what counts. However, if you are one of those people who think it is not really consummated, or that you haven't really communed with the angels, unless you and your lover climax at exactly the same moment, there are some things you can do. Learn your partner's sexual rhythm and try to match it. Get your partner talking to you during sex so that you'll have some clues. Penetrate only after she has been brought to the brink and then drive home the ball, when you know your timing is synchronized. Sometimes the only way to know is by getting your partner to clue you in, so, as I said, get her talking.

48

PLEASURE HER WITH HER OWN TOYS

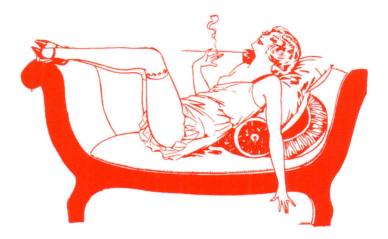

If your wife or girlfriend seems overly attached to her vibrator, don't fret. From the early Kinsey report, Psychologist Dr. Wardell Pomeroy wrote, "Many women can't seem to have an orgasm except with a vibrator." But he added, "More importantly perhaps, women may eventually be able to learn from the vibrator how to have an orgasm without it." Many men have written me over the years complaining about their lady's obsession with her vibrator and I tell them all the same thing: learn to give her orgasms equal to it and then she would never choose the fake, when she can have the real thing.

> *"Once a lover discovered my dildo in my nightstand drawer. As soon as he saw it, he decided to use it on me and I must say, he gave me a mind-blowing orgasm. I commented that I was surprised that he was so comfortable using one, as most men find them daunting to the ego. He commented, 'You can't get to the moon without a rocket ship.'"*
> —*Veronica Vera*, Miss Vera's Finishing School for Boys Who Want to Be Girls

Sexual women are generally attached to (no pun intended) and rather fond of their dildos, but what can really blow their minds is the skillful operation of that dildo in the hands of a man. So boys, instead of being jealous of her vibrator, pick it up and please her with it. You'll be surprised.

Buy her a new sex toy. Have her pick it out with you. Add to the collection now and again. Remember, variety is the spice of life.

49

CONDOMS FOR FUN?

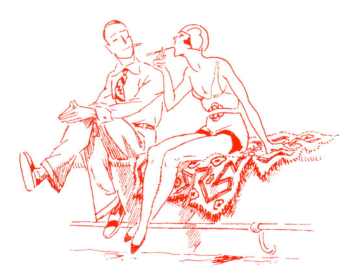

About five years ago I had a garden luncheon for a friend and we gathered all her friends, a group of pretty ladies in their mid-thirties to mid-forties, and I happened to come in from checking on my kitchen staff to hear one of them say, "It's true. Men over forty never do, and men under forty always do." When I said, "Do what?" they said, "Wear condoms." Apparently they had been comparing notes on lovers and love escapades and came to the conclusion that there is this magical, automatic dividing line and that it requires no discussion. Men under forty always have condoms and always use them. Men over forty never have condoms and never use them.

It's five years later, so I'm guessing that the under-forty crowd (now under forty-five) didn't stop using rubbers and that the over-forty-five crowd (now over fifty) didn't suddenly start.

If you are going to be promiscuous, you need to wear them. Some women report that many men today, as they age, become more interested in closing the deal on a monogamous relationship just so that they don't have to bother with the rubbers or the risk. If you don't wear them, this advice is lost on you, but if you do, be adventurous and go for variety: try the scented ones, the studded ones, the ribbed ones, the glow in the dark ones. Provide her with variety, even when it comes to condoms.

50

PROLONG THE PLAY

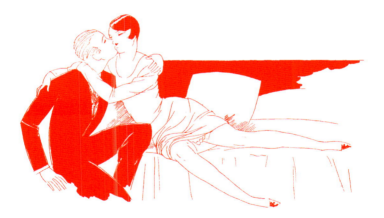

Stay in foreplay mode a long time. One thing that many men have told me is that the longer they can manage to prolong foreplay, the more time they can spend in a state of high arousal. And the longer they can delay ejaculation, the stronger and more thrilling is the orgasm when it finally happens. One tried and true example of doing this is to leisurely explore her whole body with your hands and lips (see tip #25, Think Like a Lesbian). By the time you are done with the journey, you will know which places she likes having played with. You will know where to linger, and where not to, by her responses.

Then, instead of the ever popular 69 position, lay on your stomach between her legs. You will not only enjoy a visual close up of her delectable pussy with the panoramic backdrop of her nipple-peaked breasts, but you can also caress her clitoris with your tongue. She can fondle your head and ears, but she cannot reach your cock to trigger a premature ejaculation. Meanwhile, you can thrust against the mattress to increase your own stimulation—or if it gets too exciting—be absolutely still.

In this way, you should be able to make almost any woman climax before you come yourself. Once she has her orgasm, you can slide your stiff cock into her now-soaking pussy and if you come in five strokes, she will still think you are terrific.

I have known men who can go all night having round after round of sex, without coming. They make marvelous lovers. I answered one such man whose young bride was complaining that he was too controlling of his orgasms, she was apparently getting too exhausted from the sessions. I told my reader, "As a loyal and patriotic soldier, you no doubt spend a lot of time polishing your weapon, oiling it, stripping it down, and so forth and quite rightly so! These exercises are essential for maximum efficiency in the field of battle. However, it is also important to be prepared when expecting an encounter with the enemy. When your sergeant wakes you in the morning with "Hands off cocks and on with socks!" you should obey and stay off the beat for a few days before your next sexual encounter. A period of abstinence in a healthy young man does no harm, and it may produce a level of horniness that will make you shoot your load at the dinner table, as your wife bends over to check the roast."

51

ENCOURAGE HER

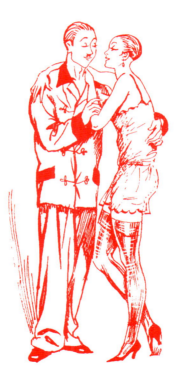

As you introduce variety into your sex life, be sure to give words of encouragement to your partner all along the way. If you want to be a great lover, then you have to provide her with great sex. If you want to provide her with great sex, you have to make it safe for her heart clit and nothing makes it safer than words of encouragement. Don't know what to say? Here are some that work, things you should feel comfortable and sincere in saying to your lady. And if you don't, then spend some time and make your own list and practice those words until they roll off your tongue.

"Damn, you are so extraordinarily beautiful."

"I can't take my eyes or hands off of you, you are so sexy."

"Being inside of you is the only place I ever want to be."

"You are so hot."

"You are so sexy."

"I want you. I have to have you."

I recently attended a wedding ceremony where the Episcopalian minister gave a most heart-warming talk to the young couple at the altar. He told the young man that there are two things that the young man should try to do every day—and it will make his marriage strong. Those two things were—number one—to make this woman (and he pointed to the bride) feel pretty and desirable and—number two—make her know that you will fight for her, at any time, in any way that life requires, that you will, indeed, fight for her. For the record, he instructed the bride that she has only one job to do and that is to treat him like a man, respect him as a man, and remind him, now and again, that he is a good man. All fodder for the heart clit.

GETTING KINKY

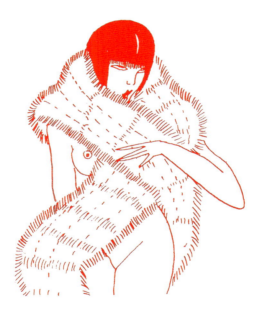

52

GETTING STARTED

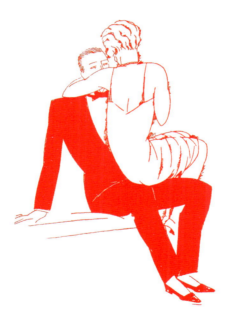

If you are in a new relationship and don't know how to suggest to your partner that you want to act out some special fantasy of yours, there are a number of subtle ways to work up to it without coming right out and saying, "Would you let me spank you?" Most women, especially, have difficulty verbalizing their fantasies, so here are some tips for working your way up to it.

We already talked about the importance of getting her talking. If she has a really hard time discussing it with you, then make her write it down for you. Ask her outright to tell you about her favorite sex dream or masturbation fantasy. Start renting erotic movies and see how the reaction to that goes. Movies are safe and couples who share a movie are expected to talk about it. Your partner may style her comments about the film in a Siskel and Ebert fashion, but you must read the body language and the delivery and you will know. Reference the listing in tip #67 for books and films that will inspire conversation.

> *"Bisexuality immediately doubles your chances for a date on Saturday night."*
> *—Rodney Dangerfield*

Books are good, but reading is a much slower process. Another way to broach a kinky subject is to tell a story you make up about a friend, who once told you he did something very erotic with his girlfriend

148

and then tell the story as you want your fantasy to go down. There's more than one way to skin that cat. And in my opinion, if you don't get to the point where you can talk about your fantasies, your sex life with this person will always be extremely limited.

Today's modern couples rely on their negotiating skills for almost all aspects of life, from purchasing a home to managing Grandma's expectations on baby-sitting night, so sex between the partners shouldn't be so different. Where sex should never be negotiable, kink should always be negotiable. A woman's willingness or ability to engage in acts that she considers kinky is highly modulated by the heart clit—the safer the heart, the higher the chances that she will play at a variety of adventures; the less trust she has, the less likely she is going to engage in anything she considers kinky.

Assuming you have made it very safe for her heart clit to allow her body clit to proceed, then negotiate for what you want. For example, if you are trying to get her to let you take erotic pictures, start out way down and off the mark with "getting a third in bed." If you know she will absolutely not do the latter, then work your way backward to the photos by making it seem like you given up a lot. All's fair in love, and war, and in the quest for mind-blowing sex.

53

PRACTICE VERBAL BONDAGE

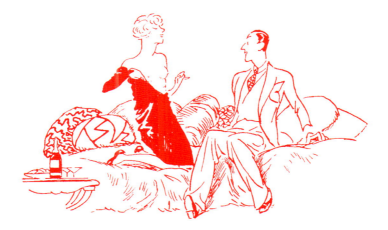

Practice verbal bondage—get your lover to give the commands, or you give the commands, but it can be very erotic to be told, "OK, put your hands here and keep them here," or "don't move," or even "be still." This is a great way to experience the fun of BDSM (bondage, domination/submission, sadism/masochism) with a new love and not have any risk of scaring her away with the paraphernalia of ropes and rigs.

In the quest for "mind-blowing" sex, never underestimate the value of words. In fact, don't underestimate the power of the voice. Voice is important. Words are important.

"It's been so long since I've had sex, I've forgotten who ties up whom."

—Joan Rivers

If you are going to involve your partner in the kinkier side of sex, then part of making it safe for her to do so, part of soothing her heart clit, is to let her know that she can make up a "safe word" and whenever she says that word, the play will stop automatically.

Most people today develop a code word to use when they are about to engage in something unusually or kinky. On the other hand, someone who has a lot of trust and faith in you might say, "No, I don't have code words. I don't believe in them." And that's because, for that person, half the fun is in knowing that there is no way out. She is having her brain clit tickled just by the thought that there is no way out and, therefore, the mere existence of a code word would spoil her fun.

54

HAVE A SPANKING GOOD TIME

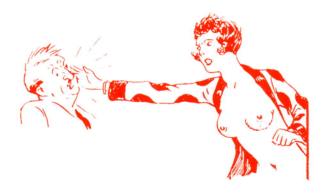

One of the theories about why people become maso-chists is that the corporal punishment they received as kids made them feel secure, secure in the bosom of the family. Getting spanked as an adult recalls that good feeling of safety as a child. My former lover refutes this by stating that she was never spanked as a child, yet she enjoyed the discipline game immensely.

Frannie came from a highly respected family whom she loved very much, but ran away from home at a young age, worked as a hooker, and did all she could to upset them. My theory is that she felt she deserved to be spanked. She certainly worked at being a bitch, in the hope that I would punish her physically, but some-times I was really sadistic and punished her by doing nothing, which drove her nuts.

> *"You don't appreciate a lot of stuff in school un-til you get older. Little things, like being spanked every day by a middle-aged women. Stuff you pay good money for later in life."*
>
> *—Elmo Phillips*

A few years ago, the Swiss Institute of Psychologi-cal Research examined why student test scores had fallen in recent years, and came up with the surpris-ing suggestion that the lower scores may be related to the banning of corporal punishment. The brain may be connected to the behind, it seems. The study of 150

154

college student volunteers found that following some swats on their backside, their ability to remember facts increased by an average of 38%.

Just because you like to paddle her ass, it doesn't make you a sadist. Wanting to experience being spanked doesn't make you a masochist, either.

For many years I had an ardent fan, a young woman from New York City, who followed me around the world. Sarah considered herself my total slave, and there was nothing she liked better than a fine spanking or whipping. At first I hesitated because I couldn't bear to hurt such a charming young woman. But I finally gave in to her constant begging, and it got so I really enjoyed giving it to her to whatever degree she wanted it. Usually, I hit her so that her buttocks turn red. As I hit her, I swore in German or Dutch. Sometimes, while her ass was still red, she would hand me a camera, and I would take pictures of her smarting backside. Because I enjoyed her company and enjoyed pleasing her, does that make me a sadist? I think not. Remember, do what makes you and your lover happy. If you enjoy what you're doing, then it's natural.

If you are going to spank your mate, make sure you have some clue about what you are doing. It doesn't matter if you use a ping pong paddle, a wooden spoon, or your hand. The erogenous zone of the bottom (in regard to spanking) is where the butt meets the top of the legs and the closer to the private parts, the better. Spanking of the vagina is fairly popular, as well.

One hard stroke, two soft, one hard, three soft—establishing a rhythm is good. Remember to read her and that the objective is to dance at her Resilient Edge of Resistance. Touching in between strokes is also good. Play and squeeze to your (and her) heart's desire. The touching is a soft contrast to the beating and the results will likely make your playmate very wet.

55

EXPERIMENT WITH HARMLESS SENSORY DEPRIVATION

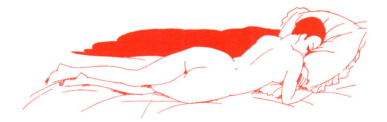

Lots of folks blindfold their mates during sex, but perhaps if you have a long stretch of time to play, you should step it up a notch. I had no idea how erotic it could be until I had an operation and lost my eyesight for forty-eight hours. It was scary. My boyfriend collected me from the clinic after the operation and, with my eyes bandaged, led me the two blocks back to the car.

The traffic seemed twice as strident as usual, and the noise made by other people on the sidewalk, the footsteps, and snatches of shouted conversation were terrifyingly loud. I had an unreasonable fear of being attacked, even though I was leaning on the strong arm of my man.

When we got home, the house was not quite as I remembered it, some distances seemed shorter and others longer, and there were far more projections and steps up and down in dangerous and unexpected places than I had ever realized. My lover prepared a wonderful meal, and although he told me afterward that his thinking was to serve me food that could be shoveled in with a spoon, it was the flavor I remember. Later, still bandaged and lightly drugged with painkillers, we made love, and the texture of his skin, the feel of his hard but invisible cock under my hand, between my lips and in my pussy, took on a new dimension.

56

ATTEND A SEX-BASED EVENT

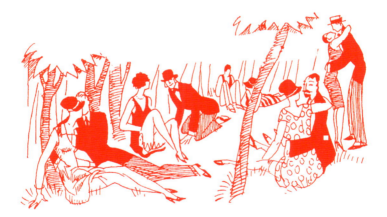

To find a swingers' party near you, go to the Internet and type in "swingers" followed by a comma and your town or city. It's that easy.

To gain acceptance to most swinger events you will need to register. Registering generally consists of sending in a photo of yourself and some money. Go there, socialize, meet people and if you feel up to it, participate. Couples tend to be pretty good about telling you what they are into and asking permission. If at any point, you feel uncomfortable, you can always say no. Also, if you want to watch and not participate, you can just tell people you are into voyeurism.

Attend an S&M workshop together. Your local S&M store often will give free workshops on how to use sex toys, care for leather products, or assume different sexual roles. These workshops can be a lot of fun to attend. I can guarantee that you will learn something new! Not only will the two of you be exposed to something new together, but then you will have a lot to talk about—and who knows where a conversation like this could lead you.

57

MAKE HOME MOVIES

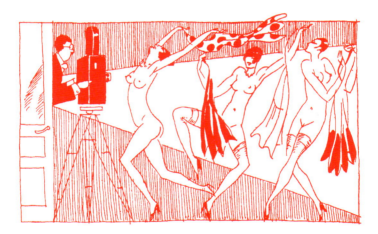

Make your own kinky movie together. Then watch it and immediately erase it. Most couples die of laughter when they watch themselves having sex. Let's face it: most people look rather silly during the act. The good news is that your partner already knows what you look like—and enjoys it with you. So, the only embarrassment you may feel is about you seeing you! However, on a few occasions, you might even find yourself looking pretty good.

Today there are many creative ways a man can use a video camera to have some fun with his woman. It's not just the filming and the playback, but the fact that the Internet provides a vast opportunity for posting materials. There are adult portals where husbands post their videos of their wives and viewers can rate them. If you are in the mood for a little harmless exhibitionism, you have all the tools today to be your own production company.

58

EXPAND THE PARTNERSHIP TO INCLUDE A THIRD PARTY

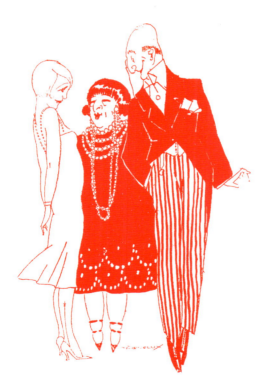

For many couples, marriage becomes dull after a few years and in order not to cheat or spend a lot of household money on porn or other alternative entertainment, many have chosen to have a third or fourth partner join in on the sexual fun. Often it starts totally harmlessly enough: the wife gets visited by the neighbor, male or female; they start chatting and eventually end with playing versions of harmless or not so harmless games. Games may be fun but then (old story) the husband walks in and catches them in on the act.

Either he gets jealous and mad, or he gets turned on and wanks off secretly, or in the end joins in on the action. Men generally like to see two women make out.

> *"The bonds of wedlock are so heavy that it takes two to carry them, sometimes three."*
> *—Alexander Dumas*

Today's "metro-men" are not nearly as homophobic as the ones I grew up with and so there is a growing tendency for hetero men to experience homosexual encounters. Though at orgies, it is still much rarer to see two men at it than two or more women.

Even very straight-laced and conservative couples sometimes arrange for a third, just to spice things up now and again. In today's liberal environment and with the advent of the Internet, it is not so uncommon for a husband to "order up" that big, tough black man for his wife to fuck on her fortieth birthday.

For those of you who are wondering, "What do we do together, exactly?" I'll give you a hint about one position that I find incredibly erotic. I call it "the sandwich screw."

It takes a very versatile, flexible, and sex-loving woman plus two good male lovers to make a perfect "sandwich." It so happens that I have experienced this kind of lovemaking, including when I had more than two men in bed with me and another woman, so it was more like an orgy, but the positioning is for two men and a woman. I had a wonderful time just watching the proceedings between the girl and the guys. One of the guys was lying on his back with my girlfriend on top of him, her back towards his stomach as he slowly penetrated her anus. Meanwhile, another guy was fucking her in the vagina. To top it all, the third guy was leaning over her face, while she sucked his cock. Believe me, that was a hot night in Toronto!

Of course, it is very important that both men have good timing and good rhythm so that their movements are synchronized. Try it on a rainy Sunday afternoon. I can't think of a better pastime.

A lot of people, men and women, crave being with two people at the same time. This is natural for people with high libidos and if you are lucky enough to be living with a very sexual person, then you should consider adding a third to the bedroom scene now and again, to satisfy that craving for her and for you.

Picking up partners together can be much more fun and exciting and successful, provided it is done naturally. For instance, you do not necessarily have to mention that you are married or partnered to each other. You could just be a good friend who likes women. This way you can share partners who suit both your tastes, and the new girl will not feel guilty about intruding on a stable marriage or relationship.

You could both participate in seducing a woman. While he chats with her, you could arrange the drinks, put on a suitable record, and lower the lights. In other words, one of you could be in charge of mood-setting and the other in charge of entertaining. You could run a nice bubble bath and set out a candle with two or three glasses of wine or champagne in the bathroom for that great moment when you all decide to step out of your clothes and frolic around in the water.

Here are some things to consider if you are planning to expand your relationship. Many men have written me after having opened their marital relationship to a third partner, a second woman. They ask how they can go about making it permanent. I tell them to ask themselves some simple questions first. Is it the open marriage you want, the threesome, or is it that you are tired of your relationship with your wife? If it is the latter, I say don't proceed. Just like you shouldn't bring children into a bad marriage, you shouldn't invite a third into a relationship permanently if that base relationship isn't good. If the relationship at home is good and the wife is willing (in other words, she likes the threesome thing too and wants to make it more permanent), then the next question to ask yourself is "Can I eat cake every day?" Any man would be happy to have a great marriage and a little extra "treat" now and again with an extra woman in the bed. You perhaps should be happy with that. After all, what happens when we eat cake every day? We get fat and our teeth fall out.

59

PARTICIPATE IN AN ORGY

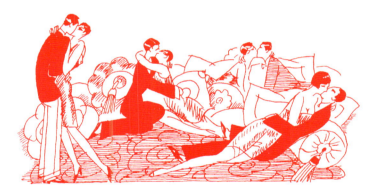

I once hosted an orgy of about thirty-six people, including a dozen or so of the old-time swingers, the rest were newcomers to the group sex game. For the first few hours any outsider would have thought that it was a normal party, because everybody kept their clothes on and didn't know how to get the ball rolling. At midnight I served some hot food and snacks and announced, half-jokingly: "Ladies and gentlemen, since this party was supposed to be an orgy, I now announce the food is ready and we can all eat or fuck, or fuck what we eat or whom we eat, but I suggest each lady start undressing at least the upper half of her partner's torso."

"The most exciting of all for a man must be when he is on his knees bent forward, supporting himself with his hands, and while one woman fondles his balls, the other sucks his cock. Just thinking about it makes me wish I was a man right now— with two chicks doing it to me, of course."
—Xaviera Hollander, Penthouse Letters, *November 1988*

And so, sometimes with effort, sometimes with finesse, the men got their shirts and sweaters and scarves peeled off. Then I announced that the men do whatever they wanted to the women. Soon there was a mutual stripping of clothing. The sexiest girls were the ones who kept on a tiny piece of clothing—a shawl, a long string of pearls, or maybe a garter belt and stockings (nobody wore bras). The amazing thing was that the new swingers who had never publicly undressed before became uninhibited in this crowd of people; the loss of inhibitions seemed to be contagious.

The next day I got many enthusiastic phone calls from people who had finally overcome their jealousy of their partner's having sex with others—as long as it remained under their close supervision and was completely sexual. Remember, your woman can call the shots on how, when, where, and just how much, but you are going to have to take that first step.

60

DO IT IN A PUBLIC PLACE

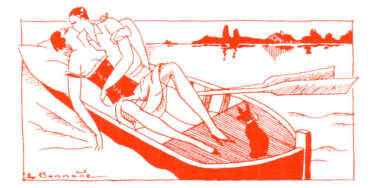

Many men have the fantasy of doing it with their girlfriends in public places, or driving down the highway with her naked body exposed, or fingering her in a highway traffic jam with a trucker watching from the next lane.

When I was in Brazil for Carnival, I happened to be riding in a car with five young Brazilian playboys. I was wearing a flimsy, low-cut dress, and since it was extremely hot, I hadn't put on a bra or panties. While two of the boys fondled and fingered me, a third had pulled down the strap of my dress to kiss my tits. We had a jolly time, especially when a local bus loaded with adults and children passed by. The banging against the glass and the screams of excitement from the windows of the bus made me have an orgasm on the spot, my pussy exposed in the wind. If your girlfriend or wife is skittish about this, then start her out slowly—with semi-private places, like the woods, and work your way up to the highways and bi-ways. (Don't be stupid though; don't try to drive and fuck at the same time. See my warning under the chapter entitled "Make 'Make-Believe' Danger.")

61

INTRODUCE HER TO VOYEURISM

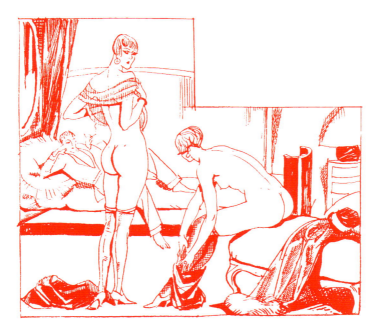

A lot of men have written me over the years about wanting to watch their wives have sex with other men. My personal theory on why a man would want to watch his wife with another man is that he is secretly bored with their physical relationships and needs reassurance that his wife is still desirable. I know dozens of marriages that actually would be strengthened if the wife could go out and get marvelously laid about once a month or even just once a year. Unfortunately, few men could handle this situation, although many of those same men would think nothing of employing a call girl for their own pleasure while on the road.

> *"Many men would like to see their wives, at least one time, being done by another man. They fantasize about it, they obsess about it, but for most, it stays in fantasy land. Most just don't know how to get there."*
>
> —*Xaviera Hollander,* Penthouse Letters, *August 1987*

Voyeurism is supposedly a masculine art, but I got enough letters over the years from women who participated and enjoyed it immensely that I know that neither sex has exclusivity on this fetish. I'm not much of a voyeur myself, but after receiving so many letters from voyeurs, I began to wonder what the thrill was.

I couldn't quite figure out the phenomenon of voyeur husbands until I tried it myself—that is, I watched my young male lover screw my young female lover. And then I understood.

I was living with a young male ballet student, and occasionally we got into things with another man or woman, or both. After a little foreplay one night, I feigned a headache and said I'd rather watch than actually participate. This surprised my lover, but he consented to make love with my girlfriend for the night, while I simply watched. Now of course I've watched him fuck other women while he's either fingered me or performed cunnilingus on me, but this was a totally different experience. I did nothing but watch. The best part was watching him shove his cock in and out of her pussy. I knew how he felt to her because I'd taken what he had so many times; a long, thin cock that could hit the spot like no other. My friend screamed with delight, and afterward she said the experience was doubly exciting because I was watching her get fucked by my own lover.

When she said that, I practically creamed in my jeans. Not only did I have to have my own lover right then and there (to show him that I was the better fuck, perhaps), but I also wanted to masturbate my friend. Somehow, I just had to feel her up where my lover, only moments before, had made love to her. Yes, sir, voyeurism can be a very erotic act and now I get it.

62

TICKLE HER FANCY

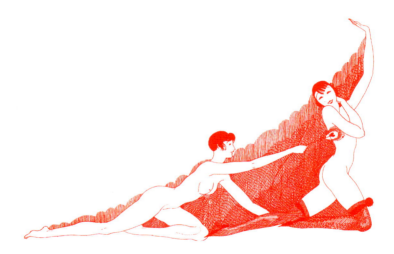

Tickling is a very common form of foreplay, and most men who have a fetish for tickling know that they are going to have to do more than get the girl in bed, whip out a feather, and say, "And now, my dear, I'm going to tickle you pink."

Try kissing her nipples, underarms, neck, ribs, belly, and feet; and after each kiss, gently tickle that part of her body with your fingers. Don't say anything—just do it! But don't linger too long over any one part of her body. Kiss and tickle her nipples for a few seconds and then move on to her ribs, and so on. That way she'll just think you're a superb lover.

If she responds positively to your tickling, you've got a ticklee on your hands, and then you can become more open about your fetish. But if the girl should say "Hey, stop that—you're tickling me!" you can always cover yourself with the line, "Oh, I'm sorry ... I was just kissing and massaging all the nooks and crannies of your beautiful body."

If this should happen and you are rejected, please don't be embarrassed or feel ashamed of your fetish. It's really very harmless and not at all uncommon. Some people are just too uptight to understand; others just don't find it erotic.

You'll discover, however, that most women find a mild degree of tickling to be very erotic.

If I were to be the tickler (versus the ticklee), I'd first tie my victim spread-eagled on my bed. Then I'd arrange a variety of props to use. For instance,

I'd certainly have a fluffy feather, a fringed tassel of silk rope, a steel hairbrush, and, of course, my long, hard fingernails. I would not limit myself to her feet. I'd also work on her armpits, flanks, and especially her sacred portal. Part of the time she'd be blindfolded so that she couldn't see which part of her body I'd tickle next.

63

IF GOLDEN SHOWERS ARE
ON YOUR LIST ...

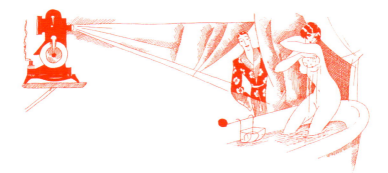

When it comes to living out golden shower fantasies, it's fair to try to enroll your partner in the game, but if after several attempts you can't convince, don't insist. Find other ways. In one of the early 2000 issues of Penthouse, they had pictures of beautiful women with their legs spread, peeing. Although it upset some readers, many more reported finding it delightfully kinky.

There's a porn video in my collection in which a well hung guy, after ejaculating in his lady's mouth, starts to pee, still with an erection. He continues for a truly remarkable length of time, while she uses his penis like a shower head, spraying her breasts, her pussy, and the rest of her body. Just goes to show that there are plenty of people who appreciate the 24-karat experience. Many women are reluctant to participate in such sports, so I recommend that if you want your wife or girlfriend to play, start slowly. Ask her to let you watch her pee and when she gets used to that, move on. Next ask her if she'll pee on you in the shower, or let you do the same to her, depending on your preference. And then remember the old adage "You can lead a horse to water, but you can't make her drink," and if after all your efforts she still doesn't want to do it, then don't.

There is nothing uncommon about a man's desire to pee on his partner. This is called "urolagnia." Hedgehogs prepare for copulation by peeing on each other. When a female mare is in heat, her urine contains a maximum concentration of female hormones. This may be one reason why some males take pleasure in sniffing female urine. Some men enjoy watching a woman urinate while squatting, as it is a symbol of her sex. Some urolagnists receive ineffable masochistic pleasure from being sprayed with urine, or even forced to drink it (I wouldn't recommend this, but I know it happens).

Urolagnia is rarer in women. I say, however, that there have been times that I have truly enjoyed taking off my suit on a beach and peeing in front of four men. As they masturbate, I quite often spray a little urine on their cocks. On occasion I have enjoyed a shot of urine against my own clitoris.

64

OTHER FINE FETISHES TO INCORPORATE INTO FOREPLAY

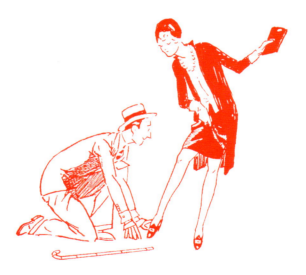

I was interviewed by a South African journalist once, while vacationing in Holland. I was staying at my mother's house. The journalist was sitting across from me on the couch as I sat in a high swivel chair. I believe my mother was making a cup of tea for us. It was a hot summer afternoon. I was very tan, wearing a light green dress and matching, high-heeled open sandals. My toenails were painted a bright red to match my fingernails.

While the man was interviewing me, I noticed that when the conversation stopped every now and then, his eyes would automatically go to my feet. I knew then that I had a **foot fetishist** in front of me.

He kept glancing at my feet and so I began to make little movements with my toes. (You might say I was toeing the line). After about ten minutes of this, the poor guy dropped his pencil and pad. He dropped to his knees and began caressing my feet. I stuck out my leg so that he could take my right foot in his hand and lick it with his tongue. It drove me wild, but at that moment my mother walked into the room. She almost dropped the tray of cookies and tea, and she threw the journalist out of her house.

Later on I explained to her that he was a harmless foot fetishist and that she had ruined a damned good interview. People have biases against foot fetishists for some reason, automatically conjuring up a vision of a man alone in a corner humping a shoe. There's no basis for it, of course, but still, men are shy of coming out and saying, "Can I suck your toes?" both for the "bad press" reason and because many women (and especially young women) are shy about experimentation.

If you're into feet, and you don't know how to tell her, take a bath with her. Under the pretense that you're soaping her body, you can play around with her feet to your heart's content. You can then find out if she likes your footwork.

*****

Lipstick is said to have first been used by the prostitutes of ancient Egypt and Phoenicia who specialized in fellatio: they highlighted their mouths to publicize their talents. Cleopatra has left a well-established reputation for fellatio. As a mark of defiance to honest women, she flaunted her vocation by reddening her lips. This vocation of Cleopatra's, which historians usually pass over in modest silence, may have had a great deal to do with her ability to captivate Caesar and Mark Anthony, despite sporting a less than average face and body.

Today the significance of lipstick is very often sexual, but it no longer indicates a particular erotic talent. A girl who wears it at an unusually early age is suspected of sexual precocity. A husband is sometimes made uneasy when his wife resumes wearing it after having abandoned it for a time.

To many men, whether cognitive of this fact or not, a lipstick-smeared mouth reminds them of the pink labia between her legs. Have you ever tried smearing lipstick on your wife's cunt lips? You should try that. And of course, don't forget to kiss it away.

*****

I have had several lovers who had a passion for performing oral sex during my **menstruation**; one of them objected strongly to my describing it as a "Dracula complex."

Many women feel extra horny just before and during their period. Wearing a diaphragm will effectively stop the blood flow, but shouldn't be counted on as birth control, since the diaphragm doesn't fit properly when the uterus swells. Some people find the idea of sex during a period distasteful, but then, some people find sex distasteful at any time. Try it and see what you both think. Tell her you can't wait to have her and she'll likely go for it.

*****

I know a lot of guys who, after a night of passion, go out into the world secretly **wearing the underpants of the woman** they have been making love to. These amateur cross-dressers all seem to have one thing in common—the desire to talk about it and explain why. Sooner or later they all confessed to me that it was because it kept them horny the whole time they were wearing them.

Predictably enough, when they told anyone else about it, whether it was the girl in question or their buddies at work, it produced an adverse result, which was a kind of shocked disapproval. Male friends accused them of being gay and many of the women found it too weird to handle. It's such a common thing with very healthy, normal, heterosexual men that I can't quite understand what all the fuss is about.

*****

In all my years running the "Call Me Madame" column for Penthouse, I heard of many fantasies—most people have them and they range from mild to truly specific out-there experiences. When trying to convince your partner to do strange things, you would be well advised to first serve your partner's fantasies. One good trick deserves another. If you can't actually do it right away, see how far you get talking about doing it. And if nothing else, sites like adultfriendfinders have made it quite easy to locate someone who shares your fetishes.

65

WAYS TO EXPLORE HER BOUNDARIES

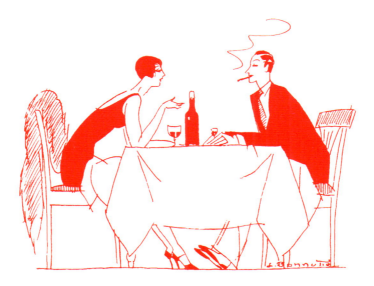

Everybody has things they won't do, even the most outrageously slutty among us. Your woman, no matter how adventurous, will have limits. The great lovers are interested in finding and knowing those limits. And the happy woman in the hands of such a man is very lucky because he will take her on an adventure that she will never forget.

Just as Barbara Carrellas recommends, when it comes to touching, play at "the Resilient Edge of Resistance." It is at the boundaries where passion lies, not within, not beyond—but at the boundaries.

Great lovers also have great patience. They know that they cannot bring a woman from no experience to the kinkiest of games without a long path leading there. If your woman has never seen a pornographic movie or magazine, if she's never masturbated, never undressed in front of a man, never was bathed or dressed by a man, never had sex in a car, never gone to a strip club, or never engaged in oral sex before, then you have a lot of time to spend just getting her through what I call "the amateur list."

Conversation is the best way to get clues to what her boundaries are, what is new to her, what might thrill and challenge her. Ask her. Have you ever purchased contraceptives? Performed a strip tease? Been photographed naked? Been caught masturbating? Watched another person masturbate? Watched a couple have sex? Been kissed by another woman? Answers to these questions will help you figure out what her experience is and that will give you clues to the starting point in the journey of discovering her boundaries. In addition, these kinds of questions make for good, stimulating conversation and story-telling. If she did ever stumble across a couple making out, you will want to know the story, and if her heart clit feels comfortable, she will tell it.

And for the not-so-faint of heart, here are some more questions that will stimulate and illuminate: Have you ever traveled over a hundred miles for the sole purpose of getting laid? Had sex with two different people in a twenty-four hour period? Cheated on your husband or boyfriend? Had sex in front of a third party? Have you ever lived in a threesome? Have you ever been to a swingers' party? Engaged in bondage? Engaged in role-play?

When finding boundaries, it's fair to use all clues and ask all kinds of questions. When actually exploring those boundaries, play at the edge where the passion lies. You need to use some sophistication and judgment and, most importantly, keep your focus on the journey and forget about the destination.

66

GAMES TO PLAY

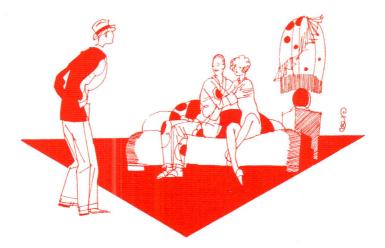

The best games to play are those that are inspired by words or actions of a fondly shared scenario, much like the private joke. The best-loved sex games that many experienced adults like to play are those they fell upon, quite by accident. If you explore her boundaries thoroughly, that journey will reveal the games you two should be playing.

> *"Most wives can't get past the idea of inviting a man over for the pure simple pleasure of having her husband watch him fuck her. Here's a suggested game to play to help ease into it. Invite one or two men that suit your wife over for 'cards.' But make it a special kind of card game and the winning and losing or the showing or not showing of particular cards equate to something—spend some time coming up with the rules together. She wins a hand, lady's choice. He wins, his choice. Maybe two pair gets him a hand-job, three of a kind a blowjob with a condom, a full house, sixty-nine, and so on. Play with it. Every gathering has their own variation; customize it to your wife's pleasure and she's certainly going to want to play."*
>
> *—Xaviera Hollander,* Penthouse Letters,
> *August 1987*

Some couples develop a private word that when heard or spoken, requires them to kiss, and not just a peck. This is perhaps more of a ritual than a game, but in the spirit of playfulness, it counts. Get a Polaroid camera and play "You Show Me Yours, I'll Show You Mine." Couples have played "Captain, May I?" in bed with satisfying results. You can take turns playing dom and sub or you can get some help from your local bookstore, as most stock board games for couples provide stimulation and excitement.

Other games to start that may lead to kinkier times:
Stage a pillow fight or wrestling match.
Visit public saunas.
Ask her to prepare a striptease for you, and you plan one for her.
Play a surprise game of hide and seek.

Get a doctor's coat and head-band with a light attached and some harmless play instruments; practice developing your "doctor" persona.

And finally, go onto one of the more popular dating portals, like adultfriendfinder, and take their purity test; both of you—and then print and compare scores and answers. Use the Internet to find erotic couples games. There are many—but be sure to retrofit them to your woman's needs and desires. Fantasies and sex games rarely come in "one size fits all."

67

READ EROTICA AND WATCH EROTIC FILMS

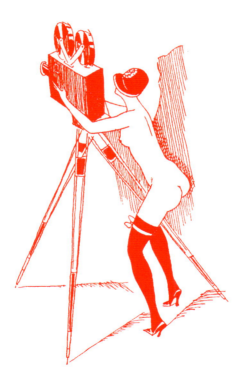

Read together. It won't do you any good if one of you, already more interested in sex than the other, goes off and reads more about it. The importance of reading and watching is in the "together" part of doing it. Here are some good books that you should take turns reading to each other. Tell your partner you want to start a new Christmas tradition that requires that she choose an interesting piece of erotica for you every year and wrap it and put it under the tree and you do the same for her. Perhaps decide on books for Christmas, films for birthdays, seeding the lawn for many years of sex-talk and sex-play.

Here are a few of my favorite choices for **books** that stimulate erotic conversation, from oldest to newest:

The Country Wife by William Wycherley (1675)
Provides plenty of material for discussion as the primary characters' attitudes on sex and marriage are challenged again and again.

Portnoy's Complaint by Philip Roth (1969)
In this classic of American literature, Alexander Portnoy has an unappeasable sexual appetite. *Life* magazine called it "a tour de force of comic and carnal brilliance."

The Sleeping Beauty Trilogy by A.N. Roquelaure (1987)
An erotic fantasy that begins with Prince Charming waking the beautiful but sleeping Beauty, and his reward for waking her, and thus saving the kingdom,

is that the King gives Prince Charming his daughter, Beauty, to be the Prince's sex slave.

The Story of O by Pauline Réage (1993)
A classic erotic novel about a dominant fashion photographer enslaving a beautiful young woman.

The Sexual Life of Catherine M. by Catherine Millet (2002) *The New York Times* calls this book "a candid, powerful and deeply intelligent depiction of unfettered sexuality"—it follows the slutty escapades of a talented and successful businesswoman.

Films are fun and faster than books, but we are talking about two different things here. Books stimulate a woman's brain clit in a very different way than movies do, so make sure you don't just focus on one or the other as a source of stimulation. Here are some of my favorites:

Lady Chatterly's Lover with Sylvia Kristel (1981)

Nine ½ Weeks with Kim Basinger (1986)

Exotica with Mia Kirshner (1994)

Striptease with Demi Moore (1996)

Breaking the Waves with Emily Watson (1996)

Secretary with Maggie Gyllenhaal (2002)

68

EXPERIMENT WITH EROTIC PROPS

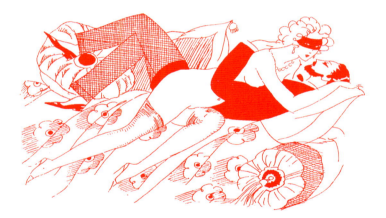

Over the years of doing the "Call Me Madame" column, I think I heard it all. Props are fun, but remember, the use of them should be aimed at enhancing the entire experience. If you happen to have some fascination with collecting pubic hairs, for example, you can't assume that she will share your interest.

Start with the usual and see how keen she is to try them:

- cigarette holders
- sexy, smeary lipstick
- rubber, leather, stiletto heels, and whips
- hair elastic used in place of a cockring—one that, when stretched, fits around the balls and is sure to get you harder, longer
- enemas
- Ben Wa balls
- remote control "egg"—ask for this at your local sex shop and they'll give you a selection, usually
- ice cubes and hot candle wax

Here's a tip that will please you both: Use a silk scarf, or better yet, silk stockings. Put them around (or on) your hands and touch her all over. The sensation will be different and titillating ... and when you are done, take the scarf, scarves, stocking or stockings, and tie them around your shaft. Make knots at the base so that when she rides you from on top, those same knots will stimulate her clit: pleasure for everyone.

69

ACT OUT ROLE-PLAY SCENARIOS

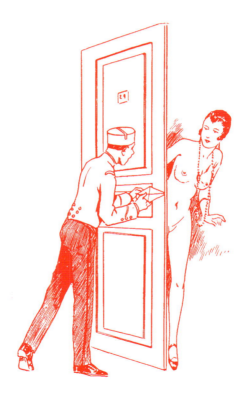

Most women will agree that the private games that blossomed out of the seed of an innocent comment are the games that tickle our brain clits the most. As an example, a friend of mine, Gina, had a girlfriend over for lunch by the pool. The friend had never met Gina's husband. She saw Gina's bare-chested husband cleaning the pool and asked Gina if he was from her pool service. Gina answered, "Yes, and I have a major crush on him."

She then poured their champagne and chatted about her fantasies of doing it with the pool dude, making sure he heard bits of it. When her husband just happened to call to her across the pool, addressing her as "Mrs. Holloway," she couldn't resist. To her friend's horror (and to Gina and her husband's great amusement), Gina walked around the pool and grabbed the pool man and engaged him in a very long kissing session. Gina returned to her friend and continued the ruse, her friend believing all the way along that the pool man was someone other than Gina's husband. Gina and her husband ended up having very good sex that afternoon, after her friend's departure, and ever after, one of their favorite games became "Playing Pool-Dude and Mrs. Holloway."

Here are a few time-tested roles to play for the idea-challenged:

- Nurse/Doctor
- Student/Teacher

- Stripper/Spectator
- Hooker/John
- Powerful Business Woman/Janitor or Male Secretary
- Bad Girl/Disciplinarian
- Disciplinarian/Bad Boy
- Secretary/Business Man
- Criminal/Police Officer (and vice versa)
- Damsel in Distress/Rescuer
- Housekeeper/House Owner

If you are going to engage in role-play, then make sure you both choose roles you like. The object here is to bring pleasure, and don't forget that. If she is totally uncomfortable playing dom to your sub, (or vice versa) you must keep searching for the kind of role-play you both like.

EPILOGUE

Over the years, many men have asked me, "Why isn't my wife/girlfriend/partner interested in sex any more?" Then, as now, the answer always goes beyond learning some new tongue trick. The answer most often has more to do with making room for sex, making sex a priority, and most importantly, giving it the excitement and respect it deserves. So, what I hope to accomplish with this book is to do more than just give you a few new tongue or finger tricks, but also give you sound advice for building a sensual relationship upon which you can continue to have mind-blowing sex for years to come.

If I missed something that you want to rail about, if I hit on something that helped you, or if you just want to be heard, please do visit my website (www.xavierahollander.com) and leave me your comments. My readers have educated me over the years and I'm still not too old to learn a new trick or two.